Journey through Anxiety and Depression

Journey through Anxiety and Depression

Dr. Jonathan Pimm

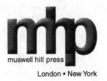

muswell hill press

London • New York

First published by Muswell Hill Press, London, 2015

www.muswellhillpress.co.uk.

British Library CIP Data available
ISBN: 978-1-908995-06-3
Printed in Great Britain

To Mie Rizig

Contents

Prologue..*xiii*

Chapter 1: Distress: Normal and Abnormal States of Mind 1
  Case Studies 1
    Stephen's Story 1
  What is Normal and What is Abnormal?.. 3
    Normal Reactions to Abnormal Circumstances.......................... 4
    Normal Reactions to Normal Circumstances 4
    Rahana's Story....'.. 5
    Abnormal Reactions to Normal Circumstances 5
    Mary Lee's Story 6
    Abnormal Reactions to Abnormal Circumstances...................... 6
  The Concept of Threshold or Subsyndromal 7
  Endogenous and Exogenous Causes (Nature Versus Nurture)......... 7
    Kevin's Story 9
  Other Physical Illnesses Causing Psychiatric Symptoms 11
    Michael's Story... 12
  Personality Issues 13
    Wayne's Story... 15
    The Psychology of Personality 15
    The Assessor 17
    Mohammed's Story: Part One 17
  The Bio-psycho-social Model 18
    Angela's Story 18
  Summary and Conclusion 19
  Neurosis and Psychosis and Comorbidity....................................... 20
  The Genetics of Depression and Other Neurotic Conditions.......... 21
  Drink and Drugs... 22
    Paul's Story... 23
  Pathways to Care.. 24
  Introduction to the Disorders... 26
    Stephen's Story: Part Two... 26

Depression 27
  Suicide and Suicidal Ideas 29
  Duration of Symptoms 31
  Number of Symptoms (Severity) 31
  Typical and Atypical Depression 32
  Stephen's Story: Part Three 32
  Dysthymia 32
  Rahanna's Story: Part Two 32
Anxiety 33
  Symptoms of Anxiety 33
  Mark's Story 35
  Stephen's Story: Part Four 36
Phobias: Specific and General 37
  Agoraphobia 37
  Galya's Story 38
  Social Phobia 38
  Jane's Story 39
Health Anxiety, Medically Unexplained Symptoms and
Somatoform Disorders 40
  Some Examples 41
  Sarah's Story 44
Physical or Mental? 44
Adjustment Disorder (Including Grief Reactions) 45
  Grief Reactions 46
Post Traumatic Stress Disorder 48
Obsessive Compulsive Disorder 49
  Obsessions 49
  Compulsions (Behaviours and Mental Acts) 50
  Stephen's Story: Part Five 50
Mixed Neurotic Disorders, Including Mixed Anxiety
and Depression 50
Bipolar Depression 52
Attention Deficit Hyperactivity Disorder in Adults 53
  Barry's Story 55
  Shareen's Story 55
Conclusions About Neurosis and Neurotic Conditions 56

Chapter 2: Treatments and Getting Help **59**
Introduction 59
Why Seek Help Now? 59
Secondary Care Assessment 63

Treatments 65
   Introduction 65
Lifestyle Considerations.. 66
   Sleep 66
   Alcohol 67
   Illicit Drugs.. 69
   Alternative Therapies... 69
   Food and Exercise 70
   Activity Scheduling 70
   Summary of Non-Traditional Treatments................................. 71
Medication.. 71
   Stephen's Story: Part Six 72
Antidepressants 72
   Side Effects of Antidepressants 76
   Withdrawal or Discontinuation Syndrome 77
   Serotonin Syndrome 77
   Suicide and the SSRIs.. 78
Anti-anxiety Drugs (Known as Anxiolytics).................................. 78
   Benzodiazepines 78
   Hypnotics.. 81
   Tryptophan.. 81
   Thyroxine.. 81
   Sodium Valproate and Other Related Anticonvulsants.............. 82
   Antipsychotics 82
   Margaret's Story 83
   Electroconvulsive Therapy (ECT).. 83
   Stimulants and Treatments for ADHD...................................... 84
Talking Treatments 86
   Counselling... 87
   Cognitive Behavioural Therapy... 88
   Psychodynamic Psychotherapy 92
   Family and Couples Therapy.. 93
Conclusion.. 94

Chapter 3: Outcomes 97
Introduction 97
The First Episode Outcome... 97
Outcomes after Repeated Episodes 99
Bipolar Depression: Treatments and Outcomes 102
Conclusion 103
And Finally 104
   Stephen's Story: Part Seven... 106

Chapter 4: Facts, Figures, Forms and Tables 107
The Professionals Involved 107
The Psychiatric Services and Teams 108
   Primary Care 108
   Secondary Care 108
The Psychiatric Assessment 110
Manuals, Questionnaires and Scales 112
   ICD 10 and DSM IV 112
   ICD-10 Diagnostic Criteria for Depression: Mild, Moderate,
   Severe 113
   DSM-IV Diagnostic Criteria for Depression 115
   NICE Guidelines 116
Questionnaires 117
   PHQ-2 117
   PHQ-9 118
   The Hospital Anxiety and Depression Scale (HADS) ... 118
   Generalised Anxiety Disorder (GAD) 119
   Adult ADHD 119
Conclusion 123

Endnotes 125
Index 131

Table of Figures

Figure 1.   Dimensions of Personality (Eysenck)   16

Figure 2.   An Example of a Timeline   65

Figure 3.   The Yerkes Dodson Curve Showing Productivity
            Against Stress   67

Figure 4.   Examples of Avoidance in Depression   71

Figure 5.   An Annotated Representation of a Synapse and
            Neuron   73

Figure 6.   Treatment Protocol for Neurotic Disorders   75

Figure 7.   The Vicious Circle of Anxiety and Depression
            (After Williams et al 2001)   80

Figure 8.   The Resolution of Depressive Symptoms in All New
            Cases (Craig 1995)   98

Figure 9.   Observed and Simulated Episode Duration Data, by
            Sex (Patten 2005)   99

Figure 10. The Neurotic Snowball (Pimm 2013)   102

Figure 11. Time to Recurrence of an Episode of Further
            Depression in People Who Had Recovered from
            Their First Bout of Unhappiness (Mueller 1999)   103

Figure 12. The Many and Varied Outcomes of Mood Disorders
            (Frank et al., 2000)   105

Figure 13. Symptoms Present in Depression   115

Figure 14. The Stepped-Care Model   117

Figure 15. Example of PHQ-2 Question   118

Figure 16. PHQ-9 Questionnaire   119

Figure 17. HADS Anxiety and Depression Scale Questionnaire   120

Prologue

Unhappiness and worry are universal. They have evolved as part of the human condition bound up with the biological responses involved in self preservation.[1] The acuteness with which any particular individual feels sadness or fear will vary even when each person faces the same difficulty. Appreciation of the distress caused by depression or anxiety is dependent upon the observer's viewpoint and dealing with such situations can be demanding and challenging.

Help in whatever form—simple reassurance, advice or medication—will in many cases provide relief. And to observe a natural smile on the face of someone previously racked with guilt and unhappiness is in itself joyful and uplifting for the medical professional or helper.

What follows is a handbook for anyone involved in the journey through these difficult conditions. It is hoped that it will provide helpful insights into the disorders as well as facts and figures about the various services, professionals and treatments available.

Throughout the book, case studies will be used to provide real-life examples of different presentations the various diseases can take. The individuals described are patients from my own practice; names and other details have been changed to protect their identities.

I would like to thank Dr Golda Ninan for her valuable assistance with this book.

JP. London. October 2013.

CHAPTER 1

Distress: Normal and Abnormal States of Mind

Case Studies

Stephen's Story

Stephen came into the surgery and stated that he had been experiencing 'total despair' for the past five months. 'It is consuming every fibre of my being', he explained. 'It is continuous, it has been totally wearing me out and it has affected my work'.

Stephen was a 49-year-old man who had been referred to me by a psychologist attached to his General Practice surgery. The psychologist had become increasingly worried about the depth of Stephen's unhappiness; she thought that he might benefit from some medication since his mood seemed to be getting worse despite several weeks of psychological talking therapy.

Stephen was a very articulate man who used rather poetic phrases to describe his mental state. He had been to university several years earlier as a mature student to study philosophy. He said he had very much enjoyed the experience and had really thrown himself into his studies.

He had been born in Bristol and his parents, who were both dead, had always been keen for Stephen to either become a lawyer or a doctor. However, in his teenage years he became rather caught up in the vibrant music scene in the area and in his words: 'went down the wrong track'.

He had two elder sisters to whom he was quite close; he was in regular telephone contact with them and visited them back in Bristol at least three times a year. They were both married and had children of their own with whom Stephen said he spent a great deal of time whenever he went back to his home city. Stephen was previously pretty much a model citizen. He was married with two children. He had been in his current job for over 10 years and never had any difficulties with his employer. He had never had a day off with any form of sickness and only ever had one or two pints of beer on a Friday night with friends or work colleagues. He had never taken any illicit drugs before and had never been involved with the police. His current problem had been developing over the past few months. He said: 'I have been breaking down for a while—but recently it has been in a league of its own'.

Stephen also explained that he had been experiencing certain periods during the day when he felt completely overwhelmed. He said that he had been obsessing, thinking over and over about things, and that he had been unable to make any decisions involving even the simplest aspects of his life; he could not, for example, decide what he should get in the supermarket when he went shopping.

He also said that he had had 'waves of anxiety' come over him during the times when he could not choose a particular course of action. He would just sit or stand motionless 'crippled by' his indecision.

He had been feeling 'absolutely exhausted' and despite going to bed early he had been waking up at about 4am. He said he was full of despair and had not been able to enjoy anything at all.

Work had been a particular source of distress to him. And he described several incidents where he had gone to someone's home to carry out an inspection of the property for asbestos and he had felt utterly despondent. He explained that he had seen the person's property all packed away in three or four suitcases and thought that this was simply the 'remnants of a life'.

In the case of Stephen, most people would probably say something was wrong. There appears to have been a dramatic change between Stephen's usual state and the way he now feels. In such a situation the difference between being well and being ill is clear. If, for example, you had recently been involved in an accident and you had broken your leg, you might go to a doctor who X-rays the bone in your thigh and then puts it in a plaster cast: the diagnosis is a fractured femur. Here the doctor is certain

If you have a runny nose, a temperature, aching limbs, a sore throat and a general feeling of listlessness and fatigue, then you probably have the flu. Here the doctor might be less certain.

In Stephen's case the diagnosis seems to be one of depression. However, in the arena of mental health (and in other branches of medicine) the distinction between being well and being ill is often particularly unclear. The reasons for the lack of clarity are many and lead to more philosophical discussions about what is normal when it comes to human emotional experiences. Feeling sad is often okay. Being anxious about a big event in your life is understandable. But being so unhappy that life feels like a never ending black hole might indicate things have gone beyond the normal state of health.

Where the boundary between mental health and mental illness is drawn depends on several factors, some relating to the sufferer and some relating the person from whom help is being sought. Others relate to society at large.

Looking at the individual first of all, it is important to put the matter in some form of context and, as far as possible, be aware of all that has gone before. In some cases, it might simply involve understanding the events in the brief period running up to the development of the problem. In other circumstances, it may be necessary to find out about events a great deal further back. In some cases again, it might be necessary to look at events taking place even before the actual patient was born; it has been shown that the environment in the womb where the baby is developing may have effects upon the behaviour of the child and subsequent adult. Further, certain conditions may be inherited from one's parents and any consideration of a patient presenting for the first time with a mental health problem should involve finding out about any illness that may run in the family.

With regard to the person from whom help is being sought (in many cases a doctor), it is well recognised that his or her beliefs, education, and personal circumstances also influence where the boundary between disease and wellness is drawn.

Finally, society and its values will have effects upon both the help seeker and the help giver; the stigma[2] of having a mental illness will often alter how the sufferer reacts and this may be specific to his or her culture. Likewise, the doctor or health professional may have prejudiced or unsympathetic ideas about patients who have mental diseases. The outcome may be even more unpredictable when both the help seeker and the health professional come from different backgrounds themselves and especially if they are both living in a foreign society with yet another set of values and prejudices; such a situation is becoming more and more common in the current global village. Such prejudices have changed with the development of more permissive societies; homosexuality, for example, was still considered to be a mental illness less than 30 years ago according to the standard psychiatric classification systems of the time.

What Is Normal and What Is Abnormal?

With any human condition that appears to be on a continuum from the so-called normal experience, there is going to be a degree of variation about where the abnormal state begins and where therefore illness is present.

Normal Reactions to Abnormal Circumstances

Sometimes people suffer terrible losses and fall victim to devastating trauma (mental and physical). A mother sees her young child becoming physically ill, a father may be involved in an accident and have to have a limb amputated, a daughter may be witness to a shocking crime or a sister may be the victim of a sexual assault. The depth and breath of human experience is almost limitless. In these cases, it might be considered normal for the individual to experience some form of mental disturbance or anguish; this might take the form of unhappiness, nightmares, feelings of anxiety and panic, constant thoughts involving the question: 'why me?' and many more problems may be found.

Not only does the actual event take many forms, which affect the outcome, but the evolution of the event over time may also vary. The trauma may have come completely out of the blue; the death of a baby, for instance, may have been unexpected and sudden. Conversely, the loss of a loved one may have been protracted and painful. Such experiences may naturally produce variations in both the length and depth of the unhappiness or other symptoms seen.

Normal Reactions to Normal Circumstances

That people react differently to abnormal circumstances will not come as any great surprise; nor then is it difficult to appreciate that people react differently to normal circumstances. Again, use of the word *normal* is imprecise, subjective and often contextual.

The dilemma in these cases is to decide whether such reactions are part of normal human experience or not. Are they (the victims) simply responding appropriately as anyone would do having been subjected to such fates?

The matter can be partly addressed by considering how disturbed the individual is and for how long they have been distressed. There are some guidelines given in the textbooks and diagnostic manuals—but these are only based upon general observations. In essence, they say, for example, with regard to the loss of a loved one, that in the majority of cases people have feelings of unhappiness and emotional numbness (sometimes known as grief), which usually last a few weeks or months. And, after such time, victims begin to put their lives back together and to slowly start resuming function somewhere near the level they were at before the trauma occurred. However, there are bound to be variations on this pattern.

The loss of a job to the dedicated hard-working employee might not be that abnormal in the scheme of things, but its impact may be very different for a variety of different reasons. He or she may become profoundly depressed with no structure, focus or goals in his or her life. The loss of the social interaction may further impact upon the individual's mood.

On the other hand, it might be that the hard-working employee is delighted at being sacked—he or she may have been so fed up with their job that it comes as a great relief to them. Perhaps the problems only arise because of spending too much time at home with a rather dominant over-bearing partner or some other domestic situation.

Take, as another example, the unqualified school leaver who has never been in more work than three months. At first sight the loss of the job to him may not be significant since he is someone who has been sacked from four jobs in as many months and who comes from a family for whom employment has been something of a rarity for several generations. However, his inability to keep the job might be utterly devastating to him. It might have been the 'final straw' that broke his psychological back and threw him into a pit of despair and hopelessness from which he could not recover.

Rahana's Story

Rahana was brought to see her doctor by her mother who said that her daughter urgently needed some 'medicine'. The patient, who was 24 years old, had been feeling unwell for about three days suffering with nausea and vomiting. She had also been going to the toilet more frequently than normal.

The patient's mother was convinced her daughter, who was due to be married in the near future, had been struck down with some form of food poisoning and simply needed an antibiotic or a similar treatment to put things right.

A few more questions strategically put to the patient during a brief physical examination prior to which the doctor had insisted the mother leave the surgery and return to the waiting area revealed that the proposed nuptials had been arranged without Rahana's consent. Tearfully she explained that she already had a boyfriend and did not want to tell her parents that she was planning her life with this man.

Abnormal Reactions to Normal Circumstances

The abnormal reaction to a normal circumstance is best illustrated with extreme examples—although, again, the use of the term *abnormal* here is contextual and open to interpretation. In this situation, one might begin to question whether or not the behaviour, response or feelings presented were true and honest; it might be the individual was deliberately misrepresenting the situation and making up the problems.

Mary Lee's Story

At the age of 34, Mary Lee suddenly developed paralysis of her arms and legs, which prevented her from standing on her feet for any length of time. She went to see her doctor, who initially referred her to a neurologist who could not find any physical cause for her difficulties and recommended that she see a psychiatrist. Her life circumstances seemed remarkably normal and unremarkable at first review. She was married to a devoted husband who had conscientiously and stoically taken two jobs in order to provide his wife and family of two young children with a good home and reasonable standard of living. They have just been away on holiday and the children have been doing well at school. The couple have lots of friends and are both well educated. After three meetings, the presence of someone else in the family home was revealed after the patient confessed to seeing a dark figure walking through her room at night. After closer questioning, it became apparent that she was not actually seeing her mother-in-law who had been staying at the family home for the past four weeks but that she was using the vision to convey the message of the presence of an unwanted guest in the house. The paralysis had developed soon after her mother-in-law's arrival and persisted for about 24 hours after her departure.

Abnormal Reactions to Abnormal Circumstances

Without too much thought it can be appreciated that the abnormal reaction (i.e., that dubbed an extreme of what might be called normal) can also been seen as a response to an abnormal circumstance.

A woman who had been raped at knife point on her way home from work one night would not be expected to turn up at the office the next day behaving as if nothing had happened.

Although, to be an abnormal reaction, it would have to be an extreme reaction—i.e., it would have to be so unexpected that a person would behave in such a way if he or she were subjected to abnormal circumstance. This situation, then, is the rarest of the four types we have discussed.

For doctors hoping to bring clarity to this confusing situation, the diagnostic manuals introduced the need for the assessor to find not only the symptoms of the disorder but also to judge the degree of 'clinically significant distress or impairment in social, occupational, or other important areas of functioning'. (APA, 2000). The aim was to separate those individuals who simply have symptoms of unhappiness or anxiety, for example, from those who are 'clinically significantly distressed' by them or who are impaired significantly in terms of their social, occupational or other important areas of functioning.

The terms are not defined, and there is no perfect test to draw the line between those who reach significance and those who do not. In effect, it was simply saying that there may be individuals who have all the signs and symptoms for a particular disorder but who carry on their lives with no apparent problems. And in these cases it is okay not to label them with a mental illness.

The Concept of Threshold or Subsyndromal

Accepting that there is a boundary between those who are mentally ill and those who are mentally healthy is to believe that people go from being well to being ill with nothing in between. Further, it implies that when people are ill they remain that way until they get better. Research on the matter has not found the reality to be so black and white.

It must be appreciated that those with mental illness develop it over a period of time; they may start with misery, they then stop enjoying themselves, they then begin to feel anxious and stop going out, they then might stop sleeping and stop eating and begin to feel that life is not worth living and start to consider ways of committing suicide. Such a situation may take days or weeks or even months to develop. And in the time before they might be considered to be suffering from a depressive disorder, for example, it is appreciated that they are below the diagnostic threshold or are *subsyndromal* for the condition. In addition, those found to be suffering from a mental disorder do not spend all their time in a constant state of illness; sometimes the intensity to which the feelings of unhappiness exist or the strength of the suicidal ideas are experienced drop below the threshold and the individual might be considered cured. Such a conclusion would be incorrect; specifically in the long-term mental disorders, previously diagnosed patients have been found to be subsyndromal or below the threshold for up to 50% of the time (see later the diagrams on long-term outcomes of mental illness).

Endogenous and Exogenous Causes (Nature Versus Nurture)

The difficulty of drawing the line between normal and abnormal is really only one part of the conundrum faced by doctors and health professionals when seeing patients with mental health or illness. The other dimension involved in the process considers the aetiology or source of the disorder once it has been decided that it is actually present.

The issue of a reaction to external situation has been discussed above, and the dilemma of deciding whether a mental illness is exogenous (being caused by factors completely outside of the body) or endogenous (being caused by factors originating only within the body) can be thought of as an extension of this.

Looking at two examples illustrating the extremes of this issue should make the concepts clearer.

At one extreme, the cause of a patient's problem could be considered totally endogenous or internal, as in the following example.

A 35-year-old woman experiences bouts of unhappiness every month. She is so unhappy that she cannot motivate herself to get out of bed and go to work. She simply stays at home not eating, not sleeping, not talking or interacting with anyone for three days before the onset of her period. And then within 24 hours she returns to her normal happy, cheerful self.

Such a case is not unusual and illustrates what would have previously been called an endogenous mood disorder arising from a change in the levels of the woman's reproductive hormones[3]. Further, it is necessary to state that everything else in the patient's life was stress free and appropriate. There were no problems before she started having periods and the problem began suddenly in her late 20s, although she had certainly been aware of mood variation that was related to her periods for many years previously.

At the other extreme, the cause of a patient's illness could be considered to be totally exogenous or external, if it really has nothing to do with the physiology or biological functioning of the individual[4]. This is illustrated by the following case.

A single mother living in south London with three children under the age of seven who has been struggling for many months to hold down a part-time job at the local supermarket has become unhappy and suicidal. She had been seen by her GP in the few weeks prior to the referral to the local psychiatric services. She had been just about coping but she reached the state of breakdown when her elderly mother, who had been helping her with the children, suddenly died.

This, then, is the other extreme where there is no clear endogenous factor but simply too many external factors that have built up over time and finally, with the death of her mother and all that entailed, the patient collapsed and developed a diagnosable disorder.

In considering the above two extreme cases, the situation appears straightforward: some cases develop due to biological features including hormonal variations, brain diseases (e.g., multiple sclerosis, or strokes or injury, or infections) whereas others develop in people subjected to terribly difficult life events and prolonged, severe mental torture or stress. In reality, however, such clear differentiation between cases is unusual. In some cases, when the disease appears to be very much biological in nature, there can be no abnormalities or pathological explanation found. And further, when the patient seems to have suffered terrible loss, with prolonged stress, and it feels that the illness is caused by external factors, an abnormal hormone level is detected on blood test.

Again, however, in many situations the case might appear to have some biological or endogenous features as well as features indicating that it has been caused by external factors like stress or loss.

Another situation that is particularly perplexing is the appearance of a clear brain disease such as multiple sclerosis where the patient develops a mental illness. It could be that the disease processes involved in the multiple sclerosis are responsible for the patient's unhappiness or it is maybe that the patient (understandably) becomes depressed and unwell because of the realisation that he or she might not be able to walk again or take part in favoured sporting activities due to the debilitating effects of the disease. In essence, these patients have developed an exogenous mental illness because of the thoughts about their endogenous disease.

The arguments involving exogenous and endogenous could be taken further if one considers the actual origin of any mental illness or disease to essentially be based within the structure of the brain. It has been shown that in certain states of mental illness, such as depression, the brain of the sufferer is indeed different from that of the non-sufferer or normal individual. The differences can only be seen with sophisticated imaging devices and these are not routinely available in clinical practice.

The debate over whether they are truly the cause of the sufferer's depressive feelings or whether they have developed these changes in the brain because of the feelings of unhappiness continues unabated. The biologist concludes that brain changes are found in all states of mental disease—some of these are easily seen and are part of recognised illnesses; others are rather non-specific and require hi-tech scanners to detect. The psychologist concludes that the changes have come about as a result of external factors impinging upon the person and that they may well be normal responses to such situations.

Kevin's Story

Kevin was a very large, well-built man in his late 50s. He had been referred by his GP after he began to experience episodes of anger and unhappiness. He had recently suffered a minor stroke, which had left him with a mild left sided weakness and some instability when walking.

His doctor, was not unduly concerned about the psychological problems and had put most of it down to his frustration about being less physically able than he had been before the stroke. When I met him, I was struck by his kindness and a strange degree of vulnerability that one would not have expected to have found it such an obviously strong and physical man. Indeed at one point during the second interview he did actually burst into tears.

The most important revelation, however, came during our third meeting when he explained that he had in fact been in prison after being convicted of the murder of a work associate. He said that he had been a rather reckless, angry young man in his 20s when the incident had occurred and that he certainly felt extremely sorry for what he had done.

He said that he had very much gone his 'own way' in life because he had come from a well-respected family; indeed, he had two brothers who were both doctors, one being a renowned surgeon.

He had been married and had three grown-up children, whom he had been purposefully avoiding because he was frightened by his anger and feared he might actually harm them. He had left the family home and rented a small flat where he felt safe because he could lock the door and avoid contact with anyone.

He said he was unhappy, he was unable to enjoy himself and found himself sitting at home in his apartment and bursting into tears while watching programmes on the television that had only the slightest hint of anything sad about them. He also said that he had become rather disorganised and that planning anything had become impossible. Previously, he explained that his friends had always relied upon him to get things done and that he had been very much the lynchpin in his social circle. He said: 'I held everything together, it was never a problem for me. I rather enjoyed being the main man, the fixer type of guy'.

When the doctor read about his previous conviction for murder, she became extremely concerned about his dangerousness and wondered whether she should continue seeing him or whether in fact he ought to be admitted under a section of the Mental Health Act to a secure psychiatric unit.[5]

Investigation of Kevin's brain with an MRI revealed damage to the frontal lobe area. The report noted the previous brain injury caused by the stroke and suggested that the frontal lobe damage had occurred around the same time, but had not been visible on the earlier image obtained using a CT scanner.

The case illustrates several important points, particularly when dealing with patients who have experienced a stroke. It is not unusual that individuals develop a clear-cut depressive illness after a cerebrovascular injury; often the actual brain damage does not affect those areas thought to be involved in the development of depressive disorders.

Clearly, it may be that patients react badly to the losses incurred as a consequence of the stroke. Kevin was previously a very physically strong man, and for him to have to walk with a stick and to be weak down one side was something he found very hard to come to terms with.

Further, the depression may develop as a consequence of the brain injury itself—although here again it may not be the direct effect of the stroke itself. Evidence has been found to suggest that patients might develop psychological difficulties through connections from the damaged area to those regions responsible for emotions and feelings.

A heightened tendency to cry (also known as pathological emotionalism) has also been described in patients after cerebrovascular disorders. Kevin might have been suffering from this phenomenon or he might have had the difficulties brought about by damage to his frontal lobe area. In cases where the frontal lobe is damaged it is often said that the patient is emotionally labile and ceases to be able to organise tasks and activities in his or her life.

Concern about his dangerousness reduced when he began to feel less irritable and his depression lifted after he was started on an antidepressant and a mood stabilising medication (sertraline and sodium valproate).

In reality, the fact that the episode of violence had occurred more than 30 years earlier, and there had been no further reports of anger or aggression up until the time of his referral, provided a degree of reassurance that he was unlikely to have posed that much risk to those he came into contact with. Further, he had such insight into his change of feelings that he had actually taken quite radical precautions against getting himself into trouble: he had left the family home and rented an apartment on his own and avoided any contact with anyone he felt might cause him to become violent.

Other Physical Illnesses Causing Psychiatric Symptoms

Diseases of the brain may present in similar ways to psychiatric illnesses. As in the case of Kevin described above, the damage caused by the stroke was directly responsible for the development of the symptoms of unhappiness and his change in behaviour.

The physical difficulties—for example, weakness of the arm or leg—can occur at the same time as the psychiatric symptoms; or they may occur before the onset of symptoms, or start after them. In some cases it might be many days, weeks or months before any clear physical difficulties are found. The patient may develop symptoms of unhappiness or anxiety or simply show subtle changes in his or her behaviour with no indication that there is any specific disease present.

Damage or illnesses directly affecting the brain are understandably important causes of psychological disturbance. Further, as a consequence or a reaction to having these illnesses, the patient may also develop depression or anxiety or other psychiatric conditions once the enormity or the seriousness of the problem he or she faces is fully appreciated.

Diseases developing in other organs outside the brain may also lead to psychiatric symptoms. Here the illness usually has its effect through a messenger, such as a hormone, or simply changes in the levels of various chemicals, vitamins or blood components will result in the patient having psychiatric symptoms.

In summary, then, many different physical illnesses affecting the brain directly or indirectly may produce problems that mimic those found in psychiatric disorders.

It is particularly important, therefore, that doctors exclude the possibility of a physical illness when they are faced with anyone with problems of depression, anxiety or any other psychological disturbances.

In reality, although most doctors will do a routine set of tests when patients first present with psychiatric difficulties, the number of times that a physical illness is found is very small. More commonly, psychological and psychiatric illnesses will present with physical symptoms for which no cause is found. See later in the book for a more detailed description of these situations.

Michael's Story

As a young man, Michael had travelled the world in the merchant navy. At the age of 67 he had been referred to me because he had begun to hit his daughter and was constantly arguing with his neighbours. He had been drinking excessively and was often found wandering about in the local area intoxicated and unkempt; he often left his flat without his shoes on and his clothes were filthy and stained.

His daughter had alerted his GP to her father's situation after she had suffered a severe cut around her eye. She had a young daughter of her own and could no longer trust her father to look after her even though he had done so without incident for several years.

Michael was a friendly, outgoing man. He was particularly proud of the fact that he had spent many years travelling the world and would often refer to his time in the navy. When I first met him, he was staggering around his apartment smelling of alcohol. He also had difficulty remembering events of the past few weeks and the reason why his daughter was no longer visiting.

During discussion of his family and previous relationships, he proudly announced that he had 13 children. He did not know their names, and neither did he know the names of their mothers (there had been 'several').

His excessive drinking and his rather aggressive, frightening manner had no doubt contributed to the belief that all his problems were due to his alcohol consumption and reluctance on the part of health professionals to get involved. However, a routine screening for physical illnesses revealed an infection of late stage syphilis.

Personality Issues

The discussion so far has focussed mainly upon the here and now or the patient's recent past, i.e., what has been happening to them in the time before they became unwell. Sometimes it is necessary to look at the patient's situation over longer periods of time, going far back into the past. The importance of such considerations is illustrated by thinking about the following two extreme examples.

Sue was always a rather shy, timid girl. Even at school she had few friends and used to run home at lunchtime to sit with her grandparents. After school she would leave class and go straight away to her mother's flat; she had little interaction with anyone outside her immediate family. She did not take any examinations and left full-time education just after her fifteenth birthday. She sat at home most of the time barely venturing out of her room.

After four years of this rather reclusive behaviour, her mother took her to the GP complaining that her daughter was depressed and needing treatment.

In this situation, the distinction between the patient's innate personality and the suspected depression is very difficult. The need to try to separate the patient's general or natural state from a more disease-based state is only important really when one considers how such a problem can be helped. Briefly, there is little point in prescribing some form of short-term treatment for entrenched, long-term problems; certainly, research evidence points to limited success with quick fixes for patients who have developed problems over many years. In essence, the longer a particular problem has been part of the person's general personality or make-up the harder it is to change and the less amenable it is to a short-term treatment.

The definition of personality involves an understanding of the pattern of thoughts, emotions and behaviours that an individual usually displays and has been displaying ever since early life in response to different situations. The terms extrovert, introvert, openness, agreeableness, conscientiousness and neurotic have been used in the description of the normal types of personality. These so-called traits can be considered in exactly the same way as mental illness and mental health in that they may be present to such an extent that they may be regarded as abnormal. But where the boundary between normal and abnormal is drawn is also difficult to determine and, again, depends upon the situation in which the individual lives.

Here the idea of 'goodness of fit' is relevant—the idea that not every type of person is suited to every type of situation. The rather tough-minded arrogant, go-getter may not fit in to the quiet, studious office environment. However, he or she might be very at home on the battlefield or the cut-throat world of newspaper journalism. Or, again, consider the placid, conscientious, obsessive type who is good at maths and who enjoys poring over spreadsheets, he or she would be well suited to life in the accounts department or the payroll section.

Appreciating such differences and variations, it can be seen that peoples' difficulties present in alternative situations and bring them into conflict in certain circumstances at various times. Further, the nature of the difficulties that arise in situations of conflict are also varied and often determined by the person's underlying personality type. For example, the tough-minded arrogant male might simply display angry outbursts in times of conflict. He or she might begin self-harming using a knife. Such a response would be unusual in the shy retiring person. He or she might present with features of anxiety and panic attacks. However, such observations are by no means universally seen. Certainly, the introverted patient is capable of violent aggressive behaviour—although generally it is not seen.

Chronic (or long-term) difficulties like unhappiness when present for many years and particularly when they develop early on in a person's life, may eventually become an individual's pervasive state; in essence, the personality becomes one dominated by unhappiness. And, further, the personality trait of introversion might deepen to such an extent that the individual is isolated, having limited social interaction and, to all intents and purposes, is unhappy. However, this does not necessarily mean that such individuals have developed unhappiness, simply that it is their personality.

And finally, there is the possibility of cases where both the personality and the unhappiness or other mental states appear together and cannot be disentangled. In these cases (which account for by far the majority of patients seen in primary care), the assessor (usually the GP) needs to decide whether or not it is a disease that can be helped with some form of treatment. The best way of doing this is to talk to someone who has known the patient for a long time; specifically in the time before their difficulties began. The aim is to obtain a complete picture of the person going as far back as possible.

Wayne's Story

Wayne was a 30-year-old man referred to see a psychiatrist because his GP wanted a second opinion about whether or not he could return to work because it was difficult to decide whether he had actually developed an illness or not. The patient said that he was too depressed to go back to his job.

He had been drinking heavily for many years and for most of his life he had been quite a tough, 'go-get-it' type. Wayne was a tough-looking man who had an intimidating quality. He had had his fair share of scrapes with the police and on several occasions been in fights where his opponent had been quite seriously injured.

He said he was depressed and that he could not motivate himself to do anything. He has been on various antidepressants but said that they had not done anything for him. He continued to binge drink every few days.

The difficulty in this case was to try and decide whether the patient really did have a depressive illness or whether the whole thing was related to problems with his personality. Or did he perhaps have problems with both depression and his personality?

The Psychology of Personality

In psychology, ideas about personality were first thought about systematically by Hans Eysenck.[6] He initially described two main types, neuroticism and extraversion/introversion, each one being on a scale or level. Everyone can be rated on each of the scales in terms of their degree of neuroticism and their degree of extraversion. The term *neuroticism* refers to a person's state of unhappiness and anxiousness. The terms *extraversion/ introversion* should be seen as two ends of a scale measuring a person's ability to be outgoing. If someone is very sociable and easy to get on with they were said to score highly on extraversion; if someone is not quite so friendly or outgoing, and are shy and cautious, they will score low on extraversion but high on the introversion end of the scale.

He later went on to add a further dimension to the introversion-extraversion/neuroticism scale. He called this dimension *psychoticism*, although it should be stressed that this term is not used in the same way as psychiatrists define it. For Eysenck, it is to do with the level of a person's mental toughness or recklessness and impulsiveness.

He further described neuroticism as being associated with feelings of anxiety, depression, and guilt, of having low self-esteem, and feeling tense, moody, worried about one's health, as if one had no control over one's life and being rather obsessive.

He thought the extraverted person was rather impulsive, active, sensation-seeking, dominant and irresponsible. And finally, he considered the psychotic person as tough-minded, masculine, achievement-orientated, unsympathetic and egocentric.

These terms, as will be seen later, have a great deal of similarity to those used in the descriptions of the individual conditions. The key thing here is to appreciate a degree of overlap between the character (personality) of an individual and the disorders that he or she might develop that would be diagnosed as depression, anxiety and other conditions.

Finally, the dimensions (extroversion/introversion-neuroticism-psychoticism) and the various types of behaviour in each one are by no means mutually exclusive. In reality, of course, most people have a bit of each one; the decision to score someone high in each of the dimensions is really based upon a general consideration of how the person behaves in a variety of different settings.

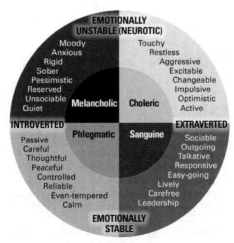

Figure 1. Dimensions of Personality (Eysenck).

The Assessor

The bias, or perhaps even bigoted views, of the assessor (for example, the psychiatrist) may have a great deal of bearing upon the outcome of the interview.

Mohammed's Story: Part One

Mohammed was a gay Bangladeshi man who had been brought up in rural area of Sylhet in North Eastern Bangladesh. He had come to the UK on a visa to study English and fell in love with a fellow student. The relationship ended and he developed depressive feelings and suicidal ideas. He was initially seen in clinic by a heterosexual, white doctor from South Africa with rather robust views about work and sexuality. The interview was an unsatisfactory one.

In Bangladesh, Mohammed had suffered a great deal of physical and mental abuse on account of his sexuality. He told me that at the age of 6 he had realised that he was different from the rest of his friends and by the time he was 13 years old, he said that he had become rather withdrawn from his school friends and concentrated only on his bookwork. He said that he had always planned to leave Bangladesh and live in a country where he could live openly as a gay man.

His difficulties were multiplied because he his visa had expired and he was living in England illegally. He could not face the possibility of returning to Bangladesh and he said that he felt he would be better off dead.

Mohammed's case can be used to usefully illustrate a simply way of looking at such problems by breaking the situation down into predisposing, precipitating and perpetuating factors contributing to the development of the current situation.

With regard to *predisposing* matters, his previous experiences as a child growing up in a homophobic society had undoubtedly led him to be a rather vulnerable, introverted, sensitive individual.

The *precipitating* factor of the relationship breakdown was important in leading Mohammed to seek help at this point.

The fear of being repatriated to Bangladesh was *perpetuating* as well as adding to his unhappiness.

The difficulties experienced by the patient may not be considered to be a disorder or a disease by the assessor. In an extreme case, an assessor may feel that he (the patient) brought it all upon himself and that he gets all that he deserves. They may feel that they would not want to attach a medical diagnosis to a situation that is essentially part of normal human experience and that the patient should seek help elsewhere.

It has long been appreciated that doctors' reactions to their patients vary depending upon the patients' ethnicity, sexuality and gender. Likewise the doctors' ethnicity, sexuality and gender have been found to have an effect upon both the patient and the outcome of the consultation. For example, it has been described that black and other ethnic minority patients will be prescribed older style antidepressants when presenting to doctors compared to non-ethnic minority patients who would more likely to receive the newer more costly medication.[7]

The Bio-psycho-social Model

Gathering information about the help-seeker is often described in terms of the biological (i.e., genetic factors including a family history of illness), psychological (i.e., important life events and circumstances) and social (i.e., the society and its values).

The term *bio-psycho-social* is used to label this type of approach. The following case illustrates the usefulness of the term.

Angela's Story

Mrs. Angela Jones was a 45-year-old housewife who requested to see a psychiatrist because she was concerned she had been taking an antidepressant for too long. In fact, she had been on medication for 'depression' for approximately 20 years. In discussion about her illness, she said that she was not in fact unhappy and that she was generally able to live a normal fulfilling life. She explained to me her concern that if she were to stop taking the antidepressant, she might suffer as she had done when she first became depressed and suicidal at the age of 17 years when she left home for the first time to go to college. She had had many further episodes of unhappiness over the following years. And on each occasion she had improved with the commencement of the antidepressant. She had also noticed that her mood tended to vary around the time of her period; she was especially unhappy and tearful in the week before her period started and then during the week after she found that she was again able to enjoy her life to the full.

Her mother had been seen by psychiatrists in the past and she (the patient) definitely remembers her mother going into a 'special hospital' for a few weeks when she was growing up.

The patient was originally from the United States and had first been diagnosed with depression by an American doctor.

At interview Mrs. Jones was a rather anxious-looking woman who made little eye contact initially, although after about twenty minutes she warmed up and appeared to be more relaxed and interactive. She had been married twice before she settled down with her current husband with whom she had two children. The family group lived together in a council-owned property, which was rather too small for them.

In reviewing Angela's case, the family history of depression in the patient's mother and the variation of the patient's mood in the context of her menstrual cycle could be considered biological factors possibly relevant for the development—or at least important in giving the patient a certain degree of susceptibility—of her mental illness. Further, the fact that she had remained well on the medication might illustrate that her illness had a strong biological component.

Her previous social circumstances might be considered psychological factors important in the development of the repeated episodes of illness.

The fact that she was first seen and diagnosed by a psychiatrist in the United States may have resulted in a woman who was only experiencing a normal reaction to a distressing situation being labelled as psychiatrically unwell. Had she been seen perhaps in the United Kingdom, she may well have just been given some supportive counselling and reassured that her experiences were perfectly understandable.

Summary and Conclusion

The differentiation between what is normal and disease is subjective. Disease is often in the eye of the patient, the beholder and in the context of society at large.

Furthermore, health professionals have drawn up guidelines and simple scales that are meant to improve the sensitivity (i.e., the ability of the doctor not to miss a single case) as well as the specificity (i.e., the ability of the doctor to be pick up only those with true illness and not those with illness that simply looks like illness) of diagnosis. As is probably appreciated, this is not an easy task.

In the discussion above, the subjects of the case histories mainly used the word *unhappiness* to describe their feelings. However, to make a particular diagnosis (e.g., depression), doctors and other health professionals look to find a collection of symptoms including an inability to enjoy life, feelings of guilt and worthlessness, suicidal ideas and poor sleep and poor appetite.

Even though an individual with a particular problem may be convinced he or she is actually ill, it is the assessor who ultimately determines whether the patient does or does not have the disorder. It is not a matter of simply the patient saying that she or he is depressed or unhappy that determines whether the doctor makes the diagnosis or not. For the diagnostic threshold to be reached there needs to be a specific depth to the problem and there needs to be a specific length of time that the symptom has been present.

Neurosis and Psychosis and Comorbidity

Drawing a distinction between mental illness and mental health is—as the preceding discussion has tried to illustrate—often not easy. However, once it has been accepted that mental illness is present and health is absent, the distinctions between the different types of mental illnesses can also become very hazy.

A major division used for many years has been to separate illnesses into those which are psychotic and those which are neurotic.

If someone is psychotic they have to have one of four features:

1. Delusions[8]
2. Hallucinations[9]
3. Disordered thoughts[10]
4. A lack of insight into their condition[11]

Any number of the different features may be present ranging from one to all four. They presence of any one of the facets distinguishes the patient from the other major category: neurosis. And, in essence, if you are mentally ill and you do not have any features of psychosis you are by definition suffering from a neurotic condition.

To appreciate the history of the term *neurosis* it is important to understand how we have reached are current way of classifying mental illnesses. The term was first used in 1772 by the Edinburgh physician William Cullen. It referred to patients who had a disorder of the nervous system without any obvious signs of a physical disease such as a fever or a rash.

In the latter part of the nineteenth century, the importance of psychological factors in the development of mental illness became recognised. And various doctors working at the time—including Sigmund Freud—focused on describing different presentations of psychological distress under the umbrella term *neurosis*.

The final and modern development of an understanding of neurotic conditions, which continues to the present time, involved the study of the extent to which the different presentations of the various conditions actually do vary. So, for example, when patients present with depression they might also have symptoms of an anxiety disorder, agoraphobia and an eating disorder as well. Which diagnostic label is actually applied depends upon which fits best. It does, however, mean that the symptoms of the other disorders are essentially ignored—a situation that, as will be shown later, may not be to the patient's advantage. Frequently patients who are depressed at the first consultation may complain more about anxiety problems or agoraphobia when they re-present at subsequent appointments. Tied up within this debate is the issue of whether the different clinical features have a common underlying cause and whether they are better treated with different medications or talking therapies.

Often the actual presentation is a result of a combinations of several neurotic conditions, personality difficulties with drug and alcohol abuse adding an additional layer of complexity to the diagnoses.

Armed with such insights, all that can be concluded is that there are some factors about the conditions that are common and that many sufferers have features at least of several of the specific conditions. Further, they may indeed have difficulties with their personality or their make-up and these may have been at least in part responsible for the development of their mental illness. Their underlying personality may have put them into a position of vulnerability from a biological point of view; their brain may not have had the necessary mental toughness to cope with certain situations. Or it might have been, for example, that because of their general make-up they had steered a pretty rocky path through life which had just been too much for them and led them to develop a mental illness.

The Genetics of Depression and Other Neurotic Conditions

Enquiry about the sensitive issue of mental health problems in other family members will frequently uncover the possibility of a strongly heritable component of the patient's depression. That genetic abnormalities or variations may be responsible at least in part for causing most psychiatric illness has been recognised for many years. The evidence for the major diseases such as schizophrenia and bipolar disorder (also known as manic depression) being passed down from generation to generation is particularly convincing. For depression and other neurotic illnesses research has undoubtedly identified a familial or inherited component that causes someone to become unwell. But this may not be found in every case and, even if it is identified, it is clear that the amount it contributes to causing a particular person's problem may vary tremendously. For some patients it may be absolutely apparent there is a strong genetic cause to their illness and the construction of a family tree tracing the disease through the different generations may be helpful.

For others, there may be no family history and it might be more important to focus on issues in the individual's personal or social life that may be responsible for causing the problems.

That genetics or heritable factors play a part in either causing or making people susceptible to developing mental illnesses is clearly important to appreciate. It is further necessary to understand that many elements of a person's make up or behaviour or indeed personality may be inherited. Specifically, it is seen that patients with more anxious or introverted personalities tend to have parents or relatives who show similar types or traits of behaviour. Such traits may develop in patients because they have simply picked them up or copied them through observation of their parents. However, it has been shown that individuals will show similar traits to their parents even when they have been separated at birth and adopted into other families where such behavioural elements were different i.e. a person may be a rather anxious, worried individual similar to his or her mother even when brought up after adoption by a confident extroverted family.

Further, it has been shown, not surprisingly, that certain personality traits – specifically those with features of anxiety and worry, i.e. introversion and nervousness will lead a person to develop depression and other neurotic illnesses more frequently.

Finally, enquiring about the drug treatments used by relatives of patients suffering from depression or any other neurotic condition may be helpful. Often the antidepressant that successfully treated one family member may be effective in the relief of symptoms for another.

Drink and Drugs

In addition to their underlying personality issues, and their more obvious features of neurotic disease, anyone involved in assessing sufferers needs to be on the look-out for drug or alcohol problems or both. People will develop features of anxiety and depression particularly if they are drinking above the recommended limits or if they are regularly using illicit drugs such as cocaine, cannabis and crack. It is surprising how often such so-called comorbid problems are overlooked in the assessment of patients with neurotic disorders, for often the anxiety and the unhappiness are fuelled by the drugs and many times they are the cause of the symptoms that have been the problem. Withdrawal from alcohol and cocaine in particular may cause symptoms that will mimic anxiety and in patients using them regularly over a longer period of time they may result in a state similar to a depressive illness. Cannabis typically causes patients to become rather suspicious and paranoid if used frequently and long term use has been associated with a state where the individual becomes apathetic and unmotivated.

Paul's Story

The atmosphere of the initial consultation had become rather uncomfortable when, after about half an hour, I began to enquire about Paul's use of illicit drugs and alcohol. He had come to see me because he had been having difficulty with feeling anxious and on edge. He had had difficulty sleeping and had been missing several days at work every week for the past few months.

He was a very pleasant, charming man in his 30s. He was of slim build and looked very fit and healthy. He had been very friendly and extremely relaxed up to the moment the issue of drug use arose.

Sheepishly he explained that he was using about a gram and a half of cocaine every day over the weekend; this essentially meant that he was taking the drug on Friday, Saturday and Sunday nights. He also said that he would drink until he could not remember—i.e., until he passed out on a couple of evenings during the week—although he re-assured me that he had not had a drink since the weekend (the day of my outpatient clinic was Thursday).

His feelings of anxiety usually became worse during the middle of the week and he had started drinking more because he said that it helped him feel less worried.

By the end of the interview it was apparent that he did not think his drug and alcohol consumption were anything to do with his difficulties either causing them directly or at least contributing to them.

At our second meeting, Paul was accompanied by his long-term partner. I had asked her to attend in order to find out whether the patient's drug and alcohol consumption had been having a detrimental effect upon their relationship. Sarah, Paul's partner of six years, was fully aware of his drug and alcohol use, and in fact she herself regularly indulged in 'taking a few lines of coke'. Both she and he thought that it had nothing to do with Paul's problems of unhappiness and anxiety. And when I delicately tried to point out to them that it might at least be making things a little worse, both became rather hostile and accused me of being 'like every other doctor' they had seen.

Sarah said: 'You are all the same you lot. You try and make out that it is all our fault. We came here looking for help and what have we got?

'If you do not want to help him, why did you see him?'

The consultation ended and they chose not to make a follow-up appointment.

Such situations are not uncommon when dealing with patients who have drug or alcohol problems. Features similar to those found in anxiety—i.e., feelings of worry, apprehension, being on edge and physical difficulties (sweating, palpitations, retching and a tremor)—are all commonly found in patients suffering from withdrawal from drugs and alcohol.

Drinking above recommended guidelines and taking illicit drugs particularly cocaine, cannabis, ecstasy and crack will also lead users to become unhappy and then possibly depressed. Taking drugs and alcohol in a binge type fashion at weekends, for example, can be particularly harmful. The individual is pretty much in a state of withdrawal from the time they stop using them; relief is only obtained with further consumption and this tends to become earlier and earlier in the working week leading to problems at the patient's place of employment.

Using drugs or alcohol in a harmful way will often lead the person to a state where they are having to drink more and take more of the illicit substance essentially just to feel 'normal'. The patient will often say that he or she only feels okay and happy when they are either drunk or under the influence of the drugs. Such a situation begins a vicious circle of decline whereby the user has to take more and more of his or her preferred substance; breaking out of this loop can be very difficult. And it is particularly problematic when the patient is not prepared to accept that the drugs or the drink are in any way involved; in the jargon of the addictions expert, the person is said to be pre-contemplative.[12]

Pathways to Care

By far and away the majority of common mental disorders are dealt with by doctors working in the primary care setting (in the UK such physicians are known as General Practitioners or GPs). The reasons why patients decide to consult their doctors at a particular point in time are varied and often difficult to work out. Their motivations to attend the surgery sometimes take a great deal of investigative work particularly when the underlying problem is a mental health one.

Many patients will not cite their anxiety or unhappiness as the reason for them seeking help. They may present with physical complaints—commonly headaches or pains of some sort; while others may clearly describe their mental health difficulties.

Further, the actual time that they present within the course of their difficulties is very variable. Some present in crises; things reach a crescendo and they literally cannot cope with their feelings any longer. They will often be very distressed in such circumstances and seek immediate consolation and treatment for their problems.

Sometimes patients will wait for many months before consulting their doctor or some other health professional about problems that have a mental health issue at their heart. The reasons for this are varied but often involve stigma—in essence a fear of what others might say about them. Further, the patient's previous experience with a health professional of matters involving mental ill health may also determine their pattern of consultation. Often they say that they feared they might not be taken seriously.

The reasons for such attitudes and beliefs and variations in consultation patterns are multiple but often involve a concern on the part of the doctor that the patient may not actually be suffering from a true illness, or that if offered treatment the patient may not comply or that the treatments on offer are particularly ineffective and therefore not really worth offering.

Mental health difficulties are not easily dealt with in the primary care setting and yet more than 90% of cases never get to see a psychiatrist or specialist. For the busy GP or family doctor the major barrier to gaining a clear understanding of the problem is a lack of time; the average consultation time in the UK is about eight minutes. Because many of these situations often involve more than one issue and more than one symptom, mental illness patients often cause frustration and despair within the doctor. Consider for example, the differences in a 20-year-old woman requesting contraceptive advice and an unemployed patient with long-standing unhappiness and anxiety with fears about leaving the house looking for help.

In the United Kingdom, GPs are usually the first health care professional seen by patients with mental health difficulties. They are helped in this monumental task by psychologists and counsellors. In Britain, the psychologists may be part of the National Health Service or they may be part of national or local charity organisations; one of the best known is MIND. Sufferers may go of their own accord to such organisations to receive talking treatment given by therapists of varying levels of experience and ability.

The GP may also recommend that the sufferer consult with therapists at these charitable organisations or he or she might suggest treatment with one of the psychologists or counsellors employed by the NHS.

Within most GP surgeries in Britain, psychologists and counsellors are employed to offer talking treatments to patients with a variety of different mental illnesses. The therapy is usually only available for a relatively short time—up to about 10 sessions held once a week, each of about an hour in duration.

For mental illnesses requiring more lengthy treatment, talking therapy is available but usually requires a referral letter from a GP and the actually sessions are normally held in a hospital.

Only about 10% of all mental health problems are seen by psychiatrists and they are usually based in the local hospital or in a satellite building in the community. Specialist services are available in larger regional centres for disorders at the more severe end of the mental illness spectrum. And referrals to these units often require both a GP letter and another assessment from a general psychiatrist.

For patients experiencing crises, services are usually based within the local general hospital where there is an Accident and Emergency Unit.[13] People requiring urgent help for mental health difficulties can go under their own steam to their nearest Accident and Emergency (A&E) Unit; or alternatively they may have decided to go to their GP initially and the doctor subsequently decided that the problem be best dealt with by a psychiatrist or a psychiatric nurse at the hospital. Patients seen at the A&E will sometimes be admitted to the nearest psychiatric unit. Alternatively, they may be referred to another department to be seen for some form of talking treatment. They may also be given medication and then seen at a later date by the psychiatrist located near their GP in the satellite building.

Recently, a new group of therapists (known as psychological wellbeing practitioners) have been introduced to many areas across England and Wales. The aim is to help patients with mental health difficulties get talking therapy as soon as possible thereby reducing the impact of the illness upon their lives. These new therapists will initially assess patients referred to them by the General Practitioner over the telephone and then decide judging on the degree of urgency and severity of the problem whether or not they need some form of talking treatment. The therapist will usually see the patient for a maximum of six sessions.

Introduction to the Disorders

Let us return again to the case of Stephen.

Stephen's Story: Part Two

As we saw, Stephen was a man in his late 40s who had been seeing a psychologist at his local surgery. He was referred to me because his difficulties had been getting worse and there were concerns for his safety because of his suicidal ideas.

His main problems were feelings of 'total despair' and tiredness. He was also complaining of unhappiness. He was unable to enjoy himself and he had been thinking that there was no way out for him and his future was bleak to the point of blackness and meaningless. He had been contemplating ending his life by driving at a concrete wall at speed or hanging himself from a tree in one of the parks in north London late at night.

Anyone reading this brief description of Stephen would probably say that he was indeed suffering from depression. And that would be correct. However, to be more precise about the diagnosis it is worth looking at the specific criteria of the condition and examining the various categories used by doctors dealing with such problems.

The problems (disorders) that will be described in this section are

Depression—both neurotic and psychotic
Anxiety—also known as generalised anxiety disorder
Phobias—specifically agoraphobia and social phobia
Somatoform disorders—health anxiety and medically unexplained symptoms
Adjustment disorder—including grief reactions
Post traumatic stress disorder (PTSD)
Obsessive compulsive disorder (OCD) and
Attention deficit hyperactivity disorder (ADHD)—specifically the problems of diagnosing the condition in adults.

Looking at all mental disorders it has been found that by far and away the most common condition is that classified as mixed anxiety and depressive disorder. This essentially means that the combination of anxiety and depression symptoms is usually found; we will explore this issue later.

The next most common condition is that of anxiety alone (22%), followed by depression (13%), then phobias (9%), obsessive compulsive disorder (6%), panic disorder (4%), and lastly those conditions where psychotic features occur (3%) of which the majority are schizophrenia and manic depressive disorder.

Depression

Unhappiness is ubiquitous. It is the fourth most common cause of disability and disease worldwide. And, according to the World Health Organisation (WHO), by the year 2020 it will be the highest ranked disease burden in most developed countries.

In the UK, depression is the third most common complaint leading patients to consult with their family doctor; the figure may vary and some researchers have found that depression may occur in up to as many as 51.5% of attendees in general practice.

Half of all women and a quarter of all men in the UK will have a depressive episode in the course of their lifetime.

People living in deprived, industrial areas are more likely to seek treatment for depression than those living in rural regions. More women suffer the problem compared to men.

The patient who complains of being 'depressed' may well be clinically[14] depressed – but simply having feelings of depression or unhappiness on their own are insufficient to fulfil the current criteria required to make a formal diagnosis of the disorder. Depression is usually only diagnosed once the sufferer has a full house of a collection of symptoms.

These symptoms are:

1. A depressed mood—the meaning of the word *mood* is not obviously apparent to many, even trainee doctors attending their first psychiatric attachments. The assessor should try to gauge the general state of the individual's happiness looking at the situation over the previous few days or even weeks. The variation from minute to minute or hour to hour that people experience to varying degrees are not generally thought of as the person's mood but are referred to as their affect. The affect may change very rapidly and is usually related to the immediate environment the individual is experiencing. Here again the clear differentiation between a depressed mood and an unhappy affect can be difficult to determine, particularly if the mood change is short and the affective change is long. In extreme cases the mood may vary rapidly from day to day and may be a mixture of unhappiness and happiness. Further, the patient may have such variation in their affect that they change from one minute to the next from being joyous and happy to either being tearful and depressed or even angry and frustrated to the point of violence. In reality, all the assessing physician can really do is to make a rough gauge of how the patient's levels of unhappiness or happiness vary.
2. A loss of interest or enjoyment—here again the degree to which the problem is present is crucial and sometimes impossible to discern.
3. A reduction in energy leading to an increased fatiguability and diminished activity.
4. A reduced ability to concentrate and pay attention to things.
5. A reduction of self-esteem and self-confidence.
6. Ideas of guilt and unworthiness.
7. Ideas or acts of self-harm or self-poisoning or suicide—see later for further discussion
8. Disturbed sleep—this may be an increase or a decrease. The decrease may occur at the beginning of the evening with so-called initial insomnia and it may occur at the end of the sleep period with so-called early morning wakening. Further, sleep may be disturbed by dreams or even flashbacks of previous traumatic events (such problems tend to

be seen when depression accompanies the presentation of Post Traumatic Stress Disorder (PTSD) and even obsessional disorders where patients have intrusive ideas, impulses and images, to be discussed below).
9. Disturbed appetite.

As the condition becomes more and more severe, the above symptoms are experienced with greater intensity and distress. The patient may become so caught up in their unhappiness that they do not even manage to 'put a brave face on it' and simply present in a slow, listless, unreactive fashion. They may lose weight and stop eating and eventually reach a point where their physical health is in grave danger.

Severe states of depression tend to develop from milder states; patients usually do not simply plunge into a life-threatening, physically debilitated state. The usual course of events is that they begin by simply feeling unhappy and then, as time passes, and the source of the upset (if there is one) continues, the unhappiness might be joined by an inability to enjoy things and then later there may be a development of feelings of guilt and problems with concentration can appear.

In some extreme cases, the patient might start believing that they are in fact dead or that parts of their body are rotting away. They may start believing that people around them are spying on them, for example, or paying them more attention when they go out travelling on public transport. Such ideas might develop further into beliefs that people are in fact talking about them; indeed, they may even reach the point where they are utterly convinced that they are the subject of strangers' conversations. Here then the patient crosses over the line between neurosis and psychosis—although, as has been emphasised several times before and will be repeated several times more, the differentiation between such states is often not clear. Psychiatrists talk about gradations of such thoughts from simply normal ideas (for example, people feeling rather uncomfortable in the presence of strangers) through to over-valued ideas (beliefs that people are possibly talking about the patient when he or she is on the bus or out in public) to psychotic delusions (for example, patients who are convinced that commuters on the bus or tube can read their mind).

Suicide and Suicidal Ideas

The matters of suicide and suicidal ideas are particular associated with depressive disorders, and anyone suffering from unhappiness should expect to be asked about such thoughts. Further, for anyone assessing a patient with a suspected depressive illness, questioning about such matters is mandatory.

It is unusual for patients to have clear plans about taking their own lives immediately. They may start simply considering that the situation would be 'better if they were not here'. They might have some vague ideas about killing themselves, which later become clear plans with full intent on the patient's part to carry them out.

The old adage about the depressed man or woman who initially complains of unhappiness and talks about death openly being the one the doctor must look out for may be important, but it has probably been given too much weight in terms of what is generally seen day to day in general practice[15].

All patients suffering from unhappiness and other symptoms of depression should be questioned about suicide. Such enquiry generates no additional risk to the patient, so there should be no hesitation in asking about such a sensitive subject. The matter is best introduced as gently as possible, and this may be done in a variety of different ways. The GP or doctor should adopt one that he or she is most comfortable with and stick to it. In reality, most patients—particularly when seeing a psychiatrist—are aware that questions about such matters are part of the process. Indeed, they may be rather miffed if they are not asked about the issue!

An assessment of ideas of suicide may be made by simply asking the patient whether he or she has ever 'felt that life was not worth living'. The question should be followed by enquiry about any plans or thoughts they have been having on the subject. Finally, the patient should be asked about previous episodes of self-harm and self-poisoning. A record of the number of times the patient has ever self-harmed and self-poisoned, the circumstances surround the event and the actions that followed it should all be documented. Any discussion about 'why?' or 'what was going through your mind at the time?' or any questions seeking to get to the bottom of the motivation for the deed will often end in confrontation and the development of feelings in the patient that the doctor or health professional thinks they were not serious about what they were doing. Clear non-judgemental questioning is the best approach, illustrated by the following sample questions.

How many times you have harmed yourself with thoughts about ending your life?

Where were you when you harmed yourself?

How many times you have taken tablets with a view to ending your life?

Where were you when you took the tablets? How many tablets did you take?

What happened after you took the tablets?

Did you leave a note or did you make any final gestures with regard to putting your things in order?
How did you get to hospital?

Generally speaking, if someone is thinking about taking his or her own life and has actually made active steps to do so then the risk involved is probably greater compared to someone who just 'wants to go to sleep and never wake up again'. For example, if someone has bought a length of rope and is planning to hang themselves or if the person has been storing up medication or has made repeated trips to the chemist to buy several boxes of paracetamol or aspirin, then the patient is to be regarded as risky.

However, to conclude that someone does not actually pose any risk just because he or she has only taken a handful of tablets or committed an act that might be viewed as rather half-hearted would be wrong. Not everyone knows that a handful of tablets of say, paracetamol, will not kill them and in the individual's mind even one tablet may have been dangerous, so taking half a dozen may have represented the ultimately fatal dose.

In general, looking at the context of the act is most important; and finding out whether or not the patient actually has an underlying mental health problem is the key. And finally, the issue of alcohol needs to be considered; many suicide attempts and completed acts are fuelled by drugs and booze.

Duration of Symptoms

Intuitively the assessor and the patient have to consider the duration of the symptoms; as might be appreciated, in the brief discussion about mood (and affect) the length of time that the troubles have been experienced is an important part of deciding whether or not someone actually has a disease. The guidelines in the UK state that the symptoms have to have been present for most days out of the previous two weeks; here again the matter of exactly how many days is most days and how many hours (or even minutes) out of each day are unclear—but such vagueness only adds to the difficulties faced by the doctor in making a definitive diagnosis that requires definitive action or treatment.

Number of Symptoms (Severity)

In addition to the time factor, or the duration that the person has been suffering with the problems of depression, the actual number of symptoms is added up to give an indication as to the severity or depth of the disease. Crudely, having four symptoms indicates a so-called 'mild' illness, between five and seven indicates a 'moderate' degree of illness and more than seven means the illness is 'severe'. The classification system used by British doctors divides the severe group into those who have psychotic features and those who do not.

Typical and Atypical Depression

Sometimes the typical biological features of depression (particularly weight loss, poor sleep and poor appetite) are reversed. The result is that sufferers may increase the amount they eat and thereby gain weight. And they may increase the amount of time they sleep spending more time in bed. There is a certain amount of fogginess about this so-called atypical depression with some debate that the problems are more part of the individual's character or personality as opposed to a neurotic condition.

Stephen's Story: Part Three

Stephen's problems became very much more worrying when he was found wandering around the town centre in a drunk and disorderly condition by the police. He had earlier had an argument with his boss and stormed out of the office saying that he never wanted to see either him or any of his colleagues ever again.

In the days before, his wife had become more concerned about her husband's behaviour; the two of them had had a terrible row (which was very unusual) and Stephen had insisted that he would be 'better off dead'.

Dysthymia

Dysthymia should be thought of as a state in which there is a chronic lowering of mood, but which fails to fulfil the criteria for a depressive disorder of either a mild or moderate severity. Suffers of dysthymia usually have periods of days or weeks when they describe themselves as well. But most of the time (often months at a time) they feel tired and depressed. Everything is an effort and nothing is enjoyed. They brood and complain. They sleep badly and feel inadequate, although they are usually able to cope with the basic demands of everyday life. Some patients in this condition were previously labelled as suffering from 'depressive personality disorder'.

Rahanna's Story: Part Two

As a child, Rahanna said she had never really been happy. Now, at the age of 32 years, she could not recall anytime in her life when she had been able to enjoy herself. She sat in the chair in the consulting room with a rather blank, expressionless face. However, she made good eye contact and was pleasant throughout the whole of the hour meeting.

She was married and had three children. Her husband, whom I met several months after my initial assessment with Rahanna, was a surprisingly happy man. He was clearly devoted to his wife and did not understand why she could not enjoy things. He explained that the children were all doing well at school. He had a good job, and they had enough money to take several holidays each year.

Sometimes, Rahanna refused to take part in family life and took herself off to her room and locked the door. Her husband often became worried that she might do something to harm herself, but her suicidal ideas were rather passive. She said: 'If I did not wake up in the morning, then that would be a blessing. I think that life is not worth it [sic]'.

She had tried various antidepressant medications and she had seen several counsellors and psychologists over the past few years. 'Nothing has helped me', she said.

Anxiety

Although more common than depression, anxiety has received much less attention from the medical profession in terms of research and clinical investigation. The majority of cases are found in women and it usually occurs in young adults aged between 20 and 29 years.

Symptoms of Anxiety

In the same way that depression has many different parts to it, the diagnosis of anxiety[16] is based upon the patient complaining of the following psychological problems or troublesome thoughts:

1. Feeling 'on edge'
2. Feeling 'as if something bad is about to happen'
3. Feeling 'worried or frightened'
4. Finding it difficult to concentrate on things
5. Finding it difficult to make a decision (in essence, indecision)
6. Feeling apprehensive about the future
7. Feeling tired
8. Feeling as if you might lose control

9. Feeling as if you might die
10. Feeling as if things around you are not real
11. Feeling as if you are not physically in the environment

Further, there may also be physical symptoms resulting in:

1. Headaches
2. Pain in many parts of the body specifically the neck, the arms and legs
3. Problems of wanting to go to the toilet a lot or feeling that you need to pass urine or faeces.
4. Problems of feeling 'butterflies in the stomach' or other feelings in the tummy like a knotted feeling
5. Difficulty with breathing—feeling out of breath or struggling for breath or gasping for air
6. Feelings of the heart beating hard in the chest or palpitations of the heart pumping in the chest
7. Feelings or pins and needles in the fingers or pain in the tips of the fingers
8. Feelings of sickness and nausea
9. Actual physical sickness and vomiting
10. Shaking of the arms and legs or excessive movement of the arms and legs (restlessness)
11. Feeling chills and hot flushes

The problem of anxiety or 'generalised anxiety disorder', as it is known, is very much the great mimic of many different physical illnesses. For example, the pains in the chest, accompanied by the shortness of breath, may look like the patient is having a heart attack. The feelings of needing to go to the toilet with feelings of nausea and vomiting might look like the patient has some form of food poisoning. The patient with the headaches and the neck stiffness might look like the patient has meningitis.

The list of the problems that symptoms associated with anxiety could be is long and involves pretty much every system in the body ranging from the nervous system to the cardiovascular (i.e., the heart and the blood vessels) to the musculoskeletal system and the respiratory system (i.e., the lungs).

Faced with such a variable and lengthy list of signs and symptoms the assessor has a tough job to get to the bottom of the problem. Further, the fact that anxiety may look like many pretty serious and life-threatening conditions, is a bit of a worry of the GP or doctor. Clearly, the first thing is too make sure there is no physical disease underlying the presentation.

Some of the physical conditions that need to be excluded are:

Endocrine disorders, including
- Hyperthyroidism—an increase in the blood levels of thyroxine or thyroid hormone.
- Hypercortisolaemia—an increase in the blood level of cortisol, which is produced by the adrenal glands on the top of the kidney.
- Hypoglycaemia—a decrease in the level of glucose in the blood. The effect can be easily felt if no food is consumed for several hours.
- Hyperparathyroidism—an increase in the levels of the parathyroid hormone.
- Phaeochromocytoma—an increase in adrenaline and similar hormones

Cardiac problems
- Particularly arrhythmias when the electrical rhythm of the heart becomes disturbed. Also similar feelings to anxiety will be experienced in the patient having a myocardial infarction (MI) or a heart attack.

Respiratory diseases
- Asthma,
- Chronic obstructive airways disease (COPD)
- Pulmonary embolus,
- Pneumonia

Vitamin deficiencies
- Especially Vitamin B12

Epilepsy
Drug and alcohol misuse, caffeine (high energy drinks) and other substances.

The majority of conditions can be excluded based on simply asking the patient a few key questions about their problems. Further, a basic physical examination and some blood tests will enable the doctor, in the majority of cases, to be confident that what he/she is dealing with is probably anxiety.

Once the diagnosis is established the real detective work can begin to try and uncover the reason why such problems have developed.

Mark's Story

The threat of redundancy for Mark, who had been in the same job for more than 25 years, and with a wife and three children at home who were dependent upon him for everything, was causing him to wake up in the middle of the night with chest pain and sweating, and with difficulty breathing. He had been to the local Accident and Emergency and was seen by a junior doctor who thought it best that he be admitted for observation overnight. In the morning the patient had been seen by the consultant who told him there was nothing wrong and that he should go home. The next day, the patient was again woken up with the same problem but decided to go to his GP in the morning; he was unable to ring his workplace to let them know why he would not be coming in that day and received a stern warning from his boss reprimanding him for not letting his workmates know where he was.

Most of the time the underlying cause for the problem is apparent after making some general enquiries about what is going on in the patient's life. And usually, without too much trouble the difficulties can be linked in the patient's mind to the physical and psychological problems he or she is having.

However, this is not always the case, particularly if the symptoms and their source have been present for a long time. Indeed, in some cases no amount of detective work will unearth the actual problem that led to the development of the anxiety in the first place; it is simply lost in the realms of time. The length of time that the patient has been suffering from the problem is very much a key indicator of how easy or how difficult it might be for the individual to return to a normal life; this aspect (known as the prognosis) will be explored in Chapter 2.

Finally, the discovery of the problem may not be sufficient to enable the patient to recover. It might be necessary for the problem to be alleviated completely before the symptoms begin to rescind. Some form of medication or psychological therapy may be necessary as well.

The differentiation of generalised anxiety disorder from more specific anxiety disorders (phobias) where the fear is actually directed towards or stems from some particular thing or situation is important for diagnostic purposes. The phobias are described in more detail below. However, in reality such clear cut boundaries between the so-called free-floating anxiety seen in generalised anxiety disorder and the phobias are rare; as we have already seen, most cases present with admixtures of several different neurotic conditions.

Re-examining the case of Stephen, it can be seen that he too had several elements of anxiety which were a problem to him.

Stephen's Story: Part Four

At an appointment with his psychologist he also said that he had had 'waves of anxiety' come over him during the times when he could not choose a particular course of action. He would just sit or stand motionless 'crippled by' his indecision.

Phobias: Specific and General

The defining attribute of phobias is the presence of fear. The individual is fearful. It may be a fear of something very specific or it may be something very general. Here the main focus of the discussion will be upon more general fears.

Specific phobias of snakes or lifts or spiders are those that tend to attract the most attention, especially from psychiatrists or health professionals. But they are not those most commonly encountered and are often not the most disabling. That is not to say that they aren't problematic to the sufferer, but encounters with snakes and spiders and even lifts are certainly not that frequent as one goes about ones everyday life. They therefore do not necessarily impact too greatly upon the sufferer's life.

By contrast, going out to the shops or meeting with strangers is pretty much an everyday occurrence; it is the phobias that concern such activities—known technically as agoraphobia and social phobia—which will be discussed here.

Agoraphobia

Agoraphobia is a fear of open spaces (the word comes from the Greek words *agora* meaning market place and *phóbos* meaning morbid fear) and tends to mean anywhere outside the home. Travelling away from the home or to any unfamiliar places will provoke feelings similar to those experienced in anxiety or generalised anxiety disorder. The sufferer may feel worried or have a sense of dread. He or she may feel apprehensive or even develop sensations that they are going to die. These psychological feelings may be accompanied by physical problems with breathing or pain or pins and needles in the hands and fingers. They may have a feeling of butterflies in the stomach or experience the urge to go to the toilet. Things might reach a point where they do in fact develop vomiting or difficulties with breathing to such an extent that they are gasping to get air.

It is not unusual that such symptoms may even develop with simply the thought of going out or the consideration of an appointment that they may have to attend sometimes several days or hours ahead.

In extreme cases the individual will experience severe anxiety sometimes labelled a panic attack (or panic disorder). The differentiation of panic disorder or panic attacks from agoraphobia is often not clear. Indeed, the two conditions are often described together. Although often patients may experience agoraphobia or simply the feelings of anxiety or fear in the absence of a full-blown episode of panic, which usually last only a few minutes (most textbooks say that the severe feelings will subside after about 20 minutes). Determining the actual length of the attack or the feelings of anxiety with the purpose of differentiating agoraphobia from panic disorder is sometimes difficult and often unhelpful. Patients will often say they have been having panic attacks when what they are probably describing is more prolonged chronic anxiety episodes; for the purposes of understanding and helping them with their problems adherence to strict diagnostic criteria is unnecessary.

Situations provoking agoraphobia may be any crowded space or area that potentially traps the sufferer. The train, the bus, the underground tube or station are all places that have been involved in patients' pathologies.

Galya's Story

Initially, Galya had been frightened only by going on the underground at rush hour. She had been pushed quite violently during rush hour one journey on her way home and decided that she could not face travelling when it was so busy. She had made special arrangements with her boss at work and had started going in later and working later so as to avoid the crowds.

Unfortunately, she had got stuck on the tube for over an hour one evening soon after she changed to her new schedule.

She had taken a few days off to try and recover. She managed to continue working for a few more months until one morning she decided that she could not face the tube journey and decided to try alternative methods of transport. She travelled partly by bus and partly on foot. She arrived more than two hours late at her office and received a verbal warning from her line manager.

She returned to the underground, but within a week she had resigned from her job and decided she was going to spend time at home looking after her teenage daughter and her husband.

Things became worse when at the local supermarket she got stuck in a long queue for the checkout. She described being unable to wait any longer and a feeling like she was about to die. She left her shopping and quickly left the store.

Social Phobia

Some degree of fear or anxiety about an important social event is pretty much universal even to the most veteran party goer just as a red flush around the neck, face and upper part of the chest can often been seen in many a seasoned public speaker or lecturer. All such reactions are perfectly normal, common and understandable. The term *social phobia* is applied when these reactions become too troublesome to the sufferer or when they fail to understand how to control such problems and are prompted to seek help from a doctor or other health professional. The other features seen as a response to the individual facing a social situation include all those previously described in anxiety or generalised anxiety disorder, which, as noted above, are the same as those seen in agoraphobia. The sufferer may develop anxiety features that reach the intensity of a panic attack and, in such a situation, will have to make his or her excuses and leave. The flee-ing of the anxiety-provoking arena may then have the appearance of the agoraphobic escaping from the crowded tube or bus.

Jane's Story

A middle-aged woman, Jane was referred by her GP to the primary care psychologist eventually got to see a psychiatrist because her description of her experiences were so involved and detailed that there was concern she was developing a serious psychotic episode. She told the psychiatrist that she felt very much like she was transported out-side of her own body and looked down upon herself whenever she had to give a briefing to the local government housing committee. She was a very clever woman who articulated her problem in such an involved, complicated way as to confuse even the most experienced health pro-fessional. Her problem was revealed when she explained that she was also a regular visitor to the lavatory before any meetings where she was invariably sick and where she had to apply large quantities of foundation to the upper part of her neck where she developed a red 'embarrassing' rash.

In both agoraphobia and social phobia the fact that the patient will begin to avoid those situations provoking the anxiety or fear unfortunately feeds into the problem. For the next time that he or she is exposed to the source of the discomfort, the reaction provoked will be even greater. Such a situa-tion then leads the patient to further avoid the fearful situations and so, the next time that they are exposed, the problems are further intensified. This growth of fear may even reach such a state that even the thought of the situation will be enough to cause the distressing reaction.

In addition to the problem of avoidance, either in physical or mental terms, the opposite situation may also arise whereby the patient cannot get the thought or fear out of his or her mind. The unfortunate term of *rumina-tion* (originating from the word used to describe animals who chew the cud[17]) describes a condition in which the patient will often be unable to get the thought of the terribly distressing experiences out of his or her mind and will keep going over it again and again. The similarity of this experience to so-called obsessions described in patients with obsessive compulsive disorder (OCD) or flashbacks or vivid memories seen in patients with post-traumatic stress disorder (PTSD) again goes to illustrate the importance of appreciating the common neurotic heritage of these conditions.

The issue of avoidance described in the phobias is exactly the same as that seen in the sufferer of PTSD.

Health Anxiety, Medically Unexplained Symptoms and Somatoform Disorders

The mind (or brain) can play tricks on us. Sometimes the physical manifestations of mental illness can be interpreted by a person with psychological distress as a serious life-threatening disease. The splitting headache resulting from stress and tension can, with a little stretch of the imagination, be thought of by the sufferer as indicating they have a brain tumour. Feelings of suffocation and difficulty with breathing brought about by anxiety can often be mistaken for a heart attack and so on. However, in reality these symptoms are part of the presentation of the disorders of anxiety and depression.

Anxiety, in particular, is a great mimic of physical problems; the list given above included pains and aches, feelings of burning, pins and needles, pressure, stomach-churning and many more.

In depression, patients often feel tired, listless, lacking in energy and weak. Furthermore, in the other neurotic conditions including agoraphobia, social phobia and obsessive compulsive disorder, which have anxiety or (fear) and depression accompanying the problems, the physical manifestations of these two disorders are commonly found as part of the presentation.

Additionally, in states of anxiety or depression, the normal physical experiences may be misinterpreted as illness; everyone, as they get older, less supple and less flexible, experiences aches and pains and stiffness of joints in many areas of the body. Set in the context of feelings of unhappiness and depression these everyday aches and pains become more and more difficult to ignore; and, indeed, the sufferer may focus upon them to such an extent that they become preoccupied with them and they become the so important or magnified in the patient's mind that they prevent them from getting on with life. Further, it is also well known that the more the individual focuses upon these difficulties the greater their significance will become. Then, further, the greater their importance is in the person's life, the more they will focus upon them. This pattern can become an escalating cycle. Later, as the unhappiness or anxiety deepens or becomes more pervasive and dominant in the individual's life, these aches and pains and other physical symptoms may become utterly disabling. They may prevent the person from walking, they may lead to constant complaints of excruciating pain and they may even have such a profound impact upon the person that they can think of nothing else in their lives.

Also, people with clear injury or disease states who experience pain or discomfort as a direct result of that identifiable disease—a common scenario being lower back pain due to some form of degenerative disorder (often called a slipped or prolapsed disc)—may then develop unhappiness or depression or some other form of mental illness. Thus, the depression or anxiety may originate either as a direct result of the patient experiencing constant aggravating pain. On top of this, the pain may keep sufferers awake at night leading to tiredness and this will then make their perception of the pain even worse. They may not be able to make love to their partner because of the pain. They may not be able to go to work because of the pain; such restrictions will make a bad situation even worse. They simply cannot do as they had done before—for example, they cannot play the sport that they loved because of the physical restriction the pain or disease state places upon them. And, as a result of the realisation of these losses, the state of unhappiness or anxiety deepens further.

Typically, one finds a combination of the two above states: the pain leads to unhappiness and the loss of function or restriction of the sufferer's life leads to even more unhappiness.

Some Examples

1. Becoming wheelchair bound because of the debilitating neurological disease multiple sclerosis put a 46-year old woman into a terrible state of unhappiness. The blow was even more devastating to her because she had been a physically fit person all her life; she had had to be because for ten years she had been a major ballerina in a famous international dance group. The mental blow of becoming disabled was an understandable cause of her unhappiness although the picture was complicated because the degenerative process of multiple sclerosis had a direct effect upon the regions of the brain involved in the perception of mood.
2. An extremely active sportswoman damaged her back during a cycling accident and was so desperate to get back on her feet again that she went directly to a private orthopaedic surgeon to have an operation.

Sadly, things did not go well and she continued to suffer with the back pain as well as weakness and paralysis of her legs. Within six months she was walking only by means of crutches and spent most of her day flat on her back in agony. A year after her operation she was confined to a wheelchair. Psychologically, she was profoundly depressed. She spent most of her time sobbing and ruminating about how bad she was feeling.

3. A young teacher who had been divorced twice in the past 10 years because she had married violent abusive men developed back pain and unhappiness, and, as a result, was unable to attend classes because she could not stay on her feet for long periods. She began isolating herself at home in her flat and broke off contact with her family. She was investigated by both the orthopaedic surgeons and the neurologists who found no abnormalities at all. Both an X-ray and an MRI scan of her lower back showed a perfectly normal spine and surrounding musculature.

Physical and mental problems (particularly unhappiness and anxiety) are intimately connected. Doctors rarely see patients who fit nicely into patterns of symptoms that they can find understandable, identifiable causes for. In fact, most patients presenting to doctors in primary care with physical problems do not have a readily identifiable cause for their difficulties.

In general practice, where such cases are common, they are simply called *medically unexplained symptoms*, (or MUSs for short). In such cases, the patient does not have a physical problem but he or she has a mental illness (usually depression or anxiety). The sufferer is in essence only focusing (or voicing concerns) about those physical manifestations of the mental illness. The more experienced GP will pick up upon the patient's distress and focus specifically upon eliciting the psychological symptoms of unhappiness or anxiety.

Sometimes the physical symptoms that the patient reports to the doctor are not easily identifiable as being caused by mental distress or psychological problems. For example, the patient may present with an epileptic seizure that looks to all intents and purposes like he or she has had a fit, and most doctors would say was clearly physical in origin. Or the patient may have developed a paralysis of the arm that looks like it is the result of suffering some form of stroke or brain damage. The patient may have developed pain in the chest with associated difficulties with breathing that looks just like a heart attack. Thus, there are some cases where patients have physical problems generated by psychological or psychiatric illness that they cannot be distinguished from the physical diseases they mimic.

Sometimes the symptoms appear like those seen in very rare illnesses. These symptoms may be so bizarre that the doctor or health professional being confronted with them may never have dealt with such a problem. These cases may get sent to highly specialised doctors who are required to decide whether the patient does actually have the very rare disease or not. For example, rare neurological illnesses may present with strange twisting movements of the body and so too may some rare psychiatric conditions.

Furthermore, the physical presentations may sometimes appear so obviously like some form of act or poor mimic of an actual illness that the patient may be thought of actually trying in some way to fake the problem.

In cases where the patient is complaining of physical symptoms originating from psychological or psychiatric illness then, the presentation may take many forms. It is then the task of the doctor or health professional to put on his or her metaphorical deerstalker and behave like a latter-day Sherlock Holmes and get to the bottom of the problem. Commonly, the actual psychiatric diagnosis in such cases is one of depression or anxiety or a mixture of the two. And usually with a little detective work the source or sources of the unhappiness or upset can be identified.

However, in about a third of all cases of so-called medically unexplained symptoms presenting in primary care, neither a physical cause nor a mental disorder is found. What, then, is the reason for such symptoms? It maybe that the patient simply could not face the psychological distress that would certainly arise if the actual reasons for being upset were to be brought out into the open; this might be interpreted in a more Freudian psychoanalytic way such that the actual psychological difficulties were converted into physical ones.[18]

An additional presentation of psychological problems that causes confusion is when patients have developed mental (or psychiatric) symptoms that look for all intense and purposes like the serious mental illnesses like schizophrenia when in fact they do not actually have such diseases. They simply have an underlying depression or anxiety that is presenting in a way that looks like they have schizophrenia. Other cases may look like a dementia-type illness or memory problem; here the unhappiness or anxiety presents with problems that are usually seen in patients who have identifiable brain damage or degeneration e.g. dementia.

So just as with patients presenting with physical symptoms where the underlying cause is anxiety or depression, serious psychiatric symptoms like hallucinations can occur in patients with an underlying anxiety or depressive disorder.

In addition, just as with some cases of medically unexplained symptoms, there are some cases of serious psychiatric symptoms (hallucinations, amnesias, or other memory difficulties) that are also found to have no clear psychological or psychiatric explanation. Such cases are only confidently diagnosed as *psychologically unexplained symptoms* (PUSs)[19] once a psychological explanation comes to light.

Sarah's Story

Sarah, a 34-year-old woman, had been complaining of seeing ghosts and tigers coming into her room at night as she lay in bed. The problem had been present for many years since her early teens. She was fully awake when the ghosts and tigers were seen and they did sometimes appear during the day. She had been fully investigated by neurologists who concluded that she did not have any form of neurological illness. Her magnetic resonance imager (MRI) brain scan revealed no abnormalities and her electro encephalogram (EEG) brain-wave tracing was normal. She was reviewed by a psychiatrist who concluded that she did not have a serious psychotic illness.

In her personal life, she was fully functioning, working for a charity in central London caring for homeless persons. She was married to a very caring, considerate man who was a famous, successful photographer, and had no children. They had no financial worries and lived in a house that they owned. She attended her outpatient appointments regularly with the psychiatrist and continued to suffer with the hallucinations.

Only after four years of regular psychotherapy did she eventually reveal to the psychologist that she had been sexually abused for several years by her uncle who used to come into her room during the night.

In the above case, the PUSs were finally explained. The explanation was clearly very painful and distressing to the patient who had kept her trauma secret for more than 15 years.

Physical or Mental?

The previous discussion will hopefully indicate that differentiation between problems in the mind and problems in the body—between the physical and the mental—is sometimes very messy.

Medically unexplained symptoms sometimes present when doctors find no physical explanation for a person's complaint. There is no underlying psychological illness, no unhappiness or anxiety—although mental illness may develop as a result of the patient suffering from a physical problem to which no explanation could be found. The physically unexplained symptom or symptoms may be painful and distressing and may result in a restriction in the patient's life, which may, in turn, also lead them to become unhappy or anxious or both.

In some cases, not only does the actual reason for the development of problem become buried but the problem presenting is not what you would have expected. Again, with reference to the above case of sexual abuse kept hidden for many years, one might have expected the patient to have been very distressed and upset, even depressed or anxious, about what had happened to her, but not that she would develop hallucinations of a tiger.

The patients with MUSs and PUSs are similar; they come with symptoms that one would not expect and they come with no explanation. A well-respected GP cleverly decided to re-brand the MUSs as 'medically unexplored stories'. In essence, he felt that sufferers of these conditions all had reasons for their problems but some remained unexplored and thus their physical presentations were unexplained.[20]

Finally, it just worth mentioning that physical problems with no explanation do rarely actually turn out to have an underlying disease and it is for this reason that doctors are advised to keep an open mind and repeat any routine investigations every so often just to make sure that nothing obvious is being missed. A word of caution here: there are two problems with doing too many investigations. Firstly, some tests might by chance just turn out to be positive even when there is nothing anything wrong (a so-called false positive). And, secondly, such focussing upon the hunt for the physical explanation may deflect attention away from the search for the important psychological cause or it may bury it even deeper within the patient's unconscious[21] mind still further; it may never allow the patient to confront or understand the underlying psychological difficulties and therefore never help them to get better.

Adjustment Disorder (Including Grief Reactions)

The discussion about abnormal and normal reactions to abnormal and normal circumstances was given to introduce the ideas that people react differently to varied situations.

An *adjustment disorder* is the term used by the diagnostic manuals to describe a variety of different states that patients get into when they faced by the usual events that life throws at us. The events are designated as normal and the reaction is abnormal.

The clinical picture may vary but includes:

1. A depressed mood
2. Features of anxiety
3. Worry (or a mixture of all three)

There may also be:

1. A feeling of being unable to cope, plan ahead or continue in the present situation
2. A degree of disability in the performance of daily routine

The individual may be liable to dramatic behaviour or outbursts of violence. In children, regressive phenomena, such as the return of bed-wetting, babyish speech or thumb-sucking, are frequently part of the symptom pattern.

The onset is usually within one month of the occurrence of the stressful event or life change and the symptoms usually resolve within six months. The International Classification of Diseases version 10 (ICD-10 manual) splits the diagnosis into seven different classes depending upon the duration:[22]

1. Adjustment disorder—a brief depressive reaction where symptoms last up to one month only
2. Prolonged depressive reaction where the disorder lasts up to two years
3. The presence of anxiety and depressive features (i.e., adjustment disorder) in a mixed anxiety and depressive reaction
4. The disturbance of other emotions including worry, tension and anger (adjustment disorder) with predominant disturbance of other emotions
5. The disturbance of conduct (adjustment disorder) with predominant disturbance of conduct which may result in aggressive or dissocial behaviour and finally
6. A presentation where both conduct and emotions are disturbed (adjustment disorder) with mixed disturbance of emotions and conduct.

Evidentially, the symptoms of an adjustment disorder are very similar to those seen in anxiety and depressive disorders. And in studies trying to differentiate adjustment disorders from depression and anxiety disorders it has been shown that any clear separation is impossible. The only way such a distinction can be made is by looking back after the event, i.e., retrospectively.

Grief Reactions

The death of someone to whom we have a level of emotional attachment is a universal experience. The psychological results are, for the most part, quite widely known; unhappiness, a sense of loss, feelings of discomfort and pangs of distress are just some of the more common experiences. Such responses are essentially normal.

Sometimes, however, more unusual things happen during the grieving process. The bereaved person might feel the presence of the individual who has died in the room. They may even say they have heard the dead person speaking or moving about. They may describe seeing brief images of him or her.

Such experiences are also considered normal. Variations from the general response seen in most people are described as abnormal and are thought of as a mental illness. Such variations are really based upon the length of time that the symptoms have continued after the death. In essence, if the grief reaction goes on too long then it is thought to be abnormal. However, such a classification fails to take into account several important variations that might surround the death and the individual experiencing the loss.

The presenting problems of the person who has suffered the bereavement may depend upon the character of the individual; as with all mental or psychological illness the underlying personality of the patient will affect how the person shows his or her emotions.

Also, the way in which the dead person met his or her end will sometimes affect the presentation of the bereaved person; if, for example, the death had been expected for several months then the friends and relatives had had time to adjust. But if the loss had been sudden and unexpected the presentation of the bereaved person may be quite different.

The quality of the relationship between the bereaved individual and the dead person will also have a bearing upon the grief reaction. Early academic explorations into the subject[23] described three different types of loss:

1. *Unanticipated* in which the bereaved individual denies that they have actually lost someone dear to them because the death was not expected or they had not prepared for it any way.
2. *Conflicted bereavement* occurs when the relationship between the deceased and the grieving individual was dysfunctional. The description given by the researchers was 'ambivalent' meaning the feelings between those involved were unclear.
3. *Chronic grief* is described where the relationship had been one where the individual was very much dependent upon the dead person, where there had been some insecurity in the way the bereaved person viewed the world.

Post Traumatic Stress Disorder

No explanation of neurosis and adjustment disorders could be complete without a brief description of post traumatic stress disorder (PTSD) since many of the symptoms found in neurotic disorders like anxiety and depression will also accompany this condition.

Considerations about PTSD have to begin by considering why it is actually labelled 'post'? This indicates that difficulties arise following an incident. PTSD is really just an extension of the normal psychological response to a very distressing experience.

The pictures or video images of people who had recently returned to the scenes of horrific genocide in the Balkans perfectly portrayed some of the normal responses human beings show when faced with extreme upset. More recently, the tragic scenes showing relatives searching among the remains of some of the towns swept away in the tsunami in Japan also give a clear picture of the immediate effects of terrible psychological trauma.

Victims appear dazed. They simply wander around among the ruins of their homes and their lives picking over the rubble and detritus. Some are eerily quiet while others are wailing loudly. All are overwhelmed by the enormity of what they are seeing and feeling; it is as if they are desperately trying to make some sense of it all and they are seeking anything that could return them to the solid ground of normality that was their lives before the experience.

These are essentially all normal responses to terrible tragedies; they are all examples of what is called an acute stress reaction by the diagnostic manuals. Such responses continue for many days and weeks, but gradually the victim begins to put things back to order and starts to live life again. They may continue to have dreams (or nightmares) about the event. They may continue to have images returning to their minds eye of what they have seen. And they may also be distressed by things that remind them of what they have experienced; watching broadcasts of similar events on the news may bring the whole raft of distress crashing back into mind. They may also deliberately avoid those things that remind them of their trauma. They may have become irritable, angry, frustrated and depressed because of their experiences; friends and family might report that their loved one has developed a tendency to snap at them as well as break down in tears seemingly for no reason.

The term PTSD is given to patients experiencing such symptoms (re-enactment phenomena such as dreams, nightmares and flashbacks, avoidance behaviour, and the agitation, anger and anxiety type problems with depression and low mood), which have continued to be a distressing problem such that the individual is unable to function. They cannot work, they cannot go out of the home and they cannot get back to anywhere near their previous normal level. They cannot put the incident behind them and move on.

The diagnostic manuals state that these problems should have started between one and six months after the initial 'shock' phase. The difficulties can continue on for an extremely variable period and may in essence 'flare up' even when they had subsided to a point where the person had returned to an apparently normal level of function.

The anger, irritability and distress type symptoms seen in patients who have gone through such traumas are clearly the same as those seen in sufferers of unhappiness and anxiety. Further, as has been already pointed out, the thoughts and images entering the mind are similar to those described as obsessional disorders (see below).

The long-term outcome of the symptoms is described in Section 2 where the longitudinal picture of all the neurotic disorders is explored in greater depth.

Obsessive Compulsive Disorder

Psychiatrists refer to obsessions as recurrent, unwanted thoughts, images and impulsive ideas. These obsessions are recognised by the patient as being self generated, and they are out of character and distressing. They may be accompanied by compulsions, which are repetitive stereotyped behaviours or mental acts driven by rules that must be applied rigidly. The rules are often intended to neutralise the anxiety or distress caused by the obsessions.

The most common symptoms of obsessive-compulsive disorder are:[24]

Obsessions

1. Fear of causing harm to someone else—the textbooks describe cases where mothers have recurrent ideas about harming their children. The ideas, however, very rarely result in any act of violence towards their loved ones.
2. Fear of harm coming to self—often the patient will talk about constant ideas of throwing himself or herself under cars or lorries.
3. Fear of contamination—commonly the sufferer thinks that they have picked up some kind of germ or infection.
4. Need for symmetry or exactness—the recurrent thought by the patient for order of things around them. It may involve furniture in a room or pencils on a desk.
5. Sexual and religious obsessions.

6. Fear of behaving unacceptably—in a public forum the individual may get the thought of shouting out some form of obscenity during a speech from an important dignitary.
7. Fear of making a mistake.

Compulsions (Behaviours and Mental Acts)

Behaviours
1. Cleaning
2. Handwashing
3. Checking
4. Ordering and arranging
5. Hoarding
6. Asking for reassurance

Mental Acts
1. Counting
2. Repeating words silently
3. Ruminations
4. 'Neutralising' thoughts

Depression will occur in 50–60% of cases of obsessive-compulsive disorder. There may also be a specific phobia identifiable and eating disorders are also found accompanying the disorder. If we look again at the case of Stephen, it can be seen that he too had elements of obsessive compulsive disorder that constantly led him to ruminate over and over again about particular aspects of his life. Such thoughts had become so overwhelming to him that they impeded him when he tried to do anything.

Stephen's Story: Part Five

At a follow-up appointment about three weeks later, Stephen also explained that he had been experiencing certain periods during the day when he felt overwhelmed every single moment. He said that he had been obsessing and thinking over and over about things and that he had been unable to make any decisions involving even simple activities.

Mixed Neurotic Disorders, Including Mixed Anxiety and Depression

In most patients presenting with neurotic symptoms there is usually a dilemma as to which specific disorder category they should be put into. It could be argued that most people at the beginning of their problem could be placed into an adjustment disorder category because very rarely do neurotic symptoms just appear out of the blue. Most frequently they are the reaction to the particular situation in which the sufferers find themselves. To differentiate between an adjustment disorder and a depressive disorder is, as already stated, an impossible task.

It might be appropriate to start trying to decide what disorder the person's symptoms could best be described as only after a suitable time period has elapsed. The question then is how long should the assessor wait before doing this? On reflection, for all the different neurotic conditions reviewed above there can be no single time frame recommended—for example, depression requires two weeks, PTSD can occur within days of an incident and an adjustment disorder can occur immediately after an event.

With regard to the issue of making a clear diagnosis when the problem seems to have features of several different neurotic conditions, the diagnostic manuals recommend that the assessor looks for the 'predominant features' and assigns the appropriate disorder label based on a sort of 'majority rule' approach. The assessment and diagnosis are usually made at the time of presentation purely and simply because it would be impractical to bring everyone back for a further in-depth interview sometime after the initial meeting. And, further, in reality the treatments for the different disorders are essentially the same.

As has already been stated, most research in this area has looked at the co-occurrence of the symptoms of depression and anxiety (generalised anxiety disorder). Indeed, a general survey of psychiatric disease found the most common disorder to be mixed anxiety and depressive disorder.[25]

In today's target-driven pressurised National Health Service in the UK, general practitioners have on average only eight minutes to see their patients. It has been found that they do not relish attendees with multitudes of symptoms, which appear to require several different diagnoses at one time. They therefore tend to pick up on the first few symptoms given to them and neglect those that might have been elicited with further exploration or questioning of the patient.

So to continue the political metaphor a little further, the 'first past the post' approach to patients with neurotic illness advises that, even though symptoms from several different diagnoses might be present in the same person, the clinician has to make the choice of just one illness and that the chosen disorder should represent the profile of the most troublesome symptoms described. So even if there are symptoms of depression, anxiety and obsessive compulsive disorder present, the diagnostician should plump for just one. For example, even though the patient might be troubled by three different disorders having seven signs and symptoms of depression, but three of anxiety and two of obsessive compulsive disorder, the diagnosis made should simply be depression. The diagnosis of a mixed anxiety and depressive disorder is one only to be made at the last resort, according to the diagnostic manuals.

Consideration of a threshold, a cut-off point, and an appreciation of subthreshold or subsyndromal presentations of the disorders has already been touched upon; such a situation should be thought of as being in constant flux with each of the different symptoms increasing or decreasing as time passes. For example, looking at the patient with OCD it can be seen that if all the different symptoms were simply to decrease in number for each disorder then the patient might be labelled subthreshold for all diagnoses. If the agoraphobic symptoms were to decrease in the agoraphobia patient then the diagnosis would become mixed anxiety and depressive disorder (MADD). If the anxiety symptoms were to decrease alone and the depressive symptoms increase then the diagnosis could easily be simple depression.

Bipolar Depression

No discussion of neurotic disorders and depression would be complete without at least a mention of the bipolar or manic depressive disorder. The diagnosis of manic depression can only be made if the patient has suffered at least one episode where the mood was elevated[26] to an excessive level and it was accompanied by other symptoms including a feeling that one's thoughts are racing, speaking fast and being full of energy. The terms *mania* and *hypomania* are differentiated by considerations about whether or not the patient's ability to function is disrupted and there are accompanying grandiose ideas that reach a level of unreality.

By definition, you cannot have manic depression unless you have had an episode of mania or hypomania; this means that you may actually have the disorder but you cannot officially diagnosed with it until you suffer a period of excessive mood elevation or irritability and the accompanying features where you lose touch with reality. It follows, therefore, that when you present with a straightforward depression or you have suffered recurrent episodes of depression you might actually have manic depression but you just have not had your first period of excessively elevated or irritable mood. Such a state is referred to as bipolar depression—it is, in essence, a manic depressive illness that has yet to have the manic upswing.

It is important therefore to be aware of such a possibility in anyone presenting with depressive symptoms, and questioning of a patient with unhappiness would be incomplete unless the health care professional had asked about the occurrence of previous episodes when the mood was elevated to an excessive level and accompanied by problems like racing thoughts, sleeplessness and feelings of being highly sexual.

In some cases the episodes of mania or hypomania may not have been brought to the attention of a doctor or another health care professional because they may not have caused the patient any problems; in fact, sometimes such periods of ultimate happiness and euphoria are treasured by the suffer and in many cases (particularly if they are towards the subsyndromal end of the spectrum) they result in the patient being extremely creative and productive both at work and at home.

Research has recently identified clues that might point towards depressed patients having a possible diagnosis of bipolar depression. These include a family history of any bipolar disorder in first-degree relatives, early age of onset, high frequency of depressive episodes, psychotic features and a period of increased energy and activity immediately preceding the depression.[27]

It is important to identify cases of bipolar depression mainly because their response to conventional antidepressant treatments is poor; indeed, such medication may actually trigger an episode of mania, which, despite what was said before about them sometimes being treasured by patients, may put individuals at great risk. The likelihood of an individual with depression developing manic depression will be discussed in chapter 3 along with treatment recommendations.

Attention Deficit Hyperactivity Disorder in Adults

A rising tide of people with difficulty focussing on their work or with problems sticking to one thing and other rather non-specific symptoms resulting from an inability to concentrate for any length of time, are presenting to health professionals.

These people often come in to the doctor's surgery saying: 'I think I've got ADHD'.

Frequently, they will have filled in an online questionnaire that has concluded they definitely have the disorder and therefore justify immediate treatment.

The reason for including a description of the disorder here is that the symptoms that lie at the heart of the sufferer thinking he or she has adult attention deficit disorder (ADHD) can be mistaken for those found in many of the neurotic disorders, particularly depression and anxiety disorders.

The subject has attracted much debate. Some do not accept it exists at all and see the whole thing as a conspiracy drummed up by the drug industry. They argue that the adult variety of the condition is not a valid concept with many people diagnosed with the disorder who never had any problems as children.

Further, they claim that more than 90% of adult patients with the diagnosis have at least one other psychiatric illness and, before treatment for ADHD is initiated, it needs to be clear that their symptoms are not caused by the comorbid problems. This is no easy task. The patients typically complain of a variety of different problems including academic impairment, an inability to focus, distractability, and disorganisation. Such difficulties are often impossible to distinguish from those seen in a variety of different psychiatric illness including many of the neurotic ones described above.

Furthermore, longstanding problematic patterns of behaviour or character difficulties are more akin to descriptions of an individual's personality (i.e., innate traits rather than pathological symptoms). The difficulties experienced by the sufferer must be seen (as with all neurotic conditions) simply as an extension of the normal. Considerations of the environment within which the person suffers the difficulties might also influence the decision to treat or not—for example, having little ability to focus upon rather dull tasks for hours on end may not suit everyone. In different situations, the same people that struggle with the dull, repetitive tasks might be described as quick witted. In places where rapid decision making is required this sort of skill would obviously be ideal.

The key symptoms to look out for are impaired attention and over activity. In children the impaired attention results in prematurely breaking off from tasks and leaving things unfinished. The overactivity leads to excessive restlessness especially in situations requiring calm. Associated features include disinhibition in social relationships, recklessness in situations involving danger and impulsive flouting of the rules (these features, it should be pointed out, are not necessary for the diagnosis nor are they diagnostic in the absence of the two cardinal features).

In adults the impaired attention persists as a lack of concentration resulting in the need to re-read materials several times, forgetting activities and appointments, losing things and losing the thread of conversations. Thoughts are unfocused and 'on the go' all the time. The overactivity may be replaced by a subjective sense of restlessness, difficulty in relaxing and settling down, and dysphoria when inactive.

Impulsivity present in children may continue into adulthood and lead to problems in teamwork, abrupt initiation and termination of relationships, and a tendency to make rapid and facile decisions without full analysis of the situation. Mood changes may be present, characterised by frequent, rapid shifts into depression or excitability, irritability and temper outbursts that interfere with personal relationships.

Barry's Story

Difficulties with his plumbing examinations had prompted Barry to seek help from his GP. He had been unable to complete the final test in his chosen profession because he just could not concentrate for long enough. He had done reasonably well at school and had left after his GCSEs at the age of 16 years. He had done a few jobs in the building trade and now at the age of 23 he had just sat his professional plumbing examinations for the first time.

He was frustrated by his inability to focus on one particular subject for longer than a few minutes at a time. His partner said that ever since she had known him he had always had difficulties with any activities that required him to sit down for prolonged periods. She said: 'He is really always on the go'. She added: 'I have always thought he had ADHD and when we saw a programme on it, both his mum and I said that's what Barry's got'.

He was clearly a bright and articulate man. He spoke quickly and when directed to answer questions managed to focus his attention without any problems. He had been referred to see an educational psychologist in his primary school, and at that stage the possibility of him being treated with medication was discussed but the idea of taking drugs did not appeal to him.

He described his mind being a bit 'like a motor' driving him to 'do stuff all the time'. He said he would go to bed at night and just lie there going over and over things until he just feel asleep exhausted.

On his second visit the clinic, I completed a recognised diagnostic questionnaire (DIVA, see chapter 4) with him, which indicated a high probability of him having the condition.

He was started on the recommended treatment and reported a vast improvement. He continued to take it for the next few months and was easily able to complete his plumbing examinations.

Such a case was clear cut. But often the true nature of the patient's difficulties is less apparent and in many cases the person attending the surgery is convinced they have a particular diagnosis, which can lead to problems.

Shareen's Story

I had been asked to see Shareen to give a second opinion as to whether she had attention deficit hyperactivity disorder (ADHD) or attention deficit disorder (ADD). She had been seen earlier in the year by another psychiatrist who felt that she did not have either disorder. He made a diagnosis of dysthymia and was convinced that she was in need of some form of long-term talking therapy.

The consultation had not gone well with my colleague because he had seen Shareen approximately five years earlier and the assessment at that stage ended after an argument. She had gone to seek help because at that time she had been convinced that she was autistic. My colleague did not feel this was the correct diagnosis at that point either and had referred Shareen to the local psychological service.

An excellent psychological formulation of the patient's problems concluded that she 'had ceased to develop mentally at around the age of 12 years.' From then on she had become 'selfish and unable to cope with the normal stresses and strains of life', stated the report.

The main difficulty Shareen wanted help with was her inability to focus on anything for longer than a few minutes. She said that her concentration was so bad that she simply could not get anything done. She was convinced she was suffering from ADHD after she read about the symptoms on the internet. She had sought help from a private psychologist who asked her to complete several questionnaires and interviewed her for approximately 50 minutes. The patient handed me a copy of the report, which concluded that Shareen had 'borderline ADD'. And it further recommended an assessment by a psychiatrist and then treatment with stimulant medication. Such a conclusion was difficult to contradict especially since Shareen had become focussed on receiving a prescription for the medication there and then.

A brief discussion about the possibility of us meeting a few weeks later and then weighting up the pros and cons of treating her with medication prompted her to reveal that she was already actually taking the stimulant dexamphetamine. She had visited a private psychiatrist three weeks ago and had been started on the drug at that consultation. We both decided that it was best she continue to seek treatment in the private sector. She explained that she had attended today because she wished to obtain the medication on an NHS prescription because it had become rather expensive getting the medication privately.

I requested that she make a follow-up appointment when she had completed her treatment with the private consultant.

Conclusions About Neurosis and Neurotic Conditions

The bio-psycho-social model helps to understand the mixture of reasons why someone might develop the symptoms of neurosis. The symptoms the patient presents with may be classifiable in one clearly defined disorder.

But more commonly the sufferer has a mixture of symptoms from an array of different disorders. The symptoms may be physical and psychological. Sometimes patients present with physical symptoms where no disease is found. In some cases these physical problems may be caused by a mental disorder. However, in other cases neither a physical disease no a mental disorder is found.

In many instances there is a clear explanation as to why the patient developed the neurotic symptoms. However, sometimes no reason for the onset of symptoms can be found. Such a situation may be difficult to appreciate because, if the problem is so distressing that it has led to the development of either physical or mental illness, one might have guessed it would be something prominent in the sufferer's mind. The concepts of repression, censorship, and the unconscious, attributed to Freud, and his model of the structure of the mind with various levels, can be used to understand the issues involved a little better.[28] Basically, the sufferer had pushed the matter to be back of his or her mind (or according to Freud the unconscious). And even though it might be a problem of extreme importance if it is kept there long enough it may become forgotten about or buried so deep that it never emerges for the clinician to appreciate.

Dealing with patients with neurotic symptoms can be extremely challenging and frustrating. It may also be very rewarding. It is the bread and butter of the work undertaken by family doctors in primary care and as such it is very important that they have an understanding of the various issues involved. Further, for anyone suffering from the problems of neurosis, appreciation of the different issues discussed above may allow them to move some way towards resolving the matter.

CHAPTER 2

Treatments and Getting Help

Introduction

When patients suffering with mental health problems seek help they have certain expectations and beliefs about what might happen. These include ideas about what the doctor might propose to help them, and whether they will get better. These ideas may be realistic and comparable to what does actually happen, or they may be so far from the truth that the patient leaves the consultation feeling utterly let down and disappointed.

Unhappiness and the other problems experienced by patients with neurotic illness are particularly prone to such divergence of patient expectation and available treatments. For the individual to have even crossed the threshold of the consulting room is quite an achievement. Often it is something that has taken a good deal of courage. It has inevitably involved the difficult step of their accepting that there might be something wrong and/or accepting the opinion of another person—possibly a husband or wife—that they should seek help.

Why Seek Help Now?

A woman in her late seventies arrives at her local surgery three days after her appointment date and is greeted by a somewhat exasperated receptionist who says to her: 'Mrs. Smith, your appointment was three days ago, why weren't you here then?' To this Mrs. Smith responds: 'How could I? Then I was sick'.

This classic anecdote illustrates the fact that reasons for patients attending their doctor are not always apparent.

Preconceptions about the course the consultation might take, in an already anxious patient, make the opening statements especially important. The doctor's first remarks may be the only ones remembered by the attendee at their initial meeting; they need to be chosen with care.

The idea that individuals are asymptomatic (i.e., free of symptoms) most of the time is incorrect; general surveys have shown that there is scarcely anyone who does not experience some symptom or the other at any given point in time. Further, the belief that the degree of seriousness of these symptoms is what motivates patients to seek help is also in many cases inaccurate. Patients will delay seeking help for many reasons including feeling guilty, ashamed, fearful, anxious, embarrassed, or because of a dislike of their physician, or because they have no one to care for their children while they attend the surgery.

Of particular relevance in psychiatric or psychological problems is the sufferer's perception of his or her diseased status, cultural factors and stigma. The fear of being given a psychiatric label will depend upon several factors including the patient's past experience of healthcare, knowledge of someone else's experience of the system and their treatment by the local community, and beliefs about the treatments available (fear of side effects and of the development of dependency on the drugs are of particular importance specifically when considering issues of compliance).[29]

Conversely, many patients attend their doctor with seemingly minor difficulties. Their illness behaviour could be thought of as abnormal unless one considered the context of their presentation.[30]

Sickness affords patients certain privileges including the right to be exempted from normal activity (such as work), being regarded as in need of care, and not being blamed for having caused the illness. However, the privileges also carry with them certain obligations: firstly, to seek medical advice; and, secondly, to want to get well as quickly as possible.[31] This process also involves the doctor treating them; for example, the physician is given the privilege of being able to examine the patient physically and psychologically as well as having professional autonomy and authority. In such a position the doctor has a duty to be objective and neutral (e.g., not to judge patients' behaviour on moral grounds) and to use his or her professional skills for the benefit of the patient and the community.

The impact of the individual doctor on patients' consulting behaviour should not be underestimated. Many patients are willing to wait for several days before they can see a particular doctor. In some cases the original problem may have diminished or even resolved itself by the time they get to see their physician yet they may still decide to attend.

Many patients have spent days and weeks building up to the consultation. They have worked out exactly what they want to say and how they are going to say it. They may enter the room and simply blurt out all their symptoms in the first few minutes. Or they may be cautious and shy to speak about issues they have been bottling up.

The severity of the patient's distress and his or her beliefs about the extent of the disability caused by the disease are the most important determinants of perceiving a need for help.

That patients tend to present in times of crises, or when they just 'cannot stand it anymore' (the feelings, stress, tension, etc.) is well recognised. It is important to appreciate that such a crisis is often not the right time to begin digging around in the more distressing parts of the sufferer's life. Instead, it may be a good time to offer a supportive, understanding base from which the patient may then begin the long process of trying to heal. Patients may also have unrealistic expectations about what can be achieved by their doctor. They may be seeking a 'quick fix' solution and may be rather disappointed when they don't get it.

So what happens when the unhappy or anxious patient first goes to his or her doctor? Research has shown that patients often fear revealing feelings of unhappiness. They are sensitive to even the slightest cues from their doctors that might indicate disinterest or impatience with such complaints. In extreme cases, the worry about a negative reaction from the doctor may be so great that patients will mask their symptoms to ensure they do not upset their physician and thus disrupt the consultation. Therefore, a proactive effort on the part of the doctor is often required in the management of psychological disorders in primary care.

The Hungarian born physician Michael Balint pioneered studies examining the interactions between doctors and their patients. A statement appearing in his classic text, "The doctor, his patient and the illness", published in 1964 stated: 'The ability to listen is a new skill, necessitating a considerable though limited change in the doctor's personality'.[32]

The current vogue of a patient-centred clinical method is one most suited to assessing and treating attendees with psychological and psychiatric complaints. However, the issue of consultation length is one that continues to cause problems for both patients and doctors. Physicians protest about a lack of time for the increasing number of tasks involved in routine consultations and they report greater satisfaction with surgeries if they have enough time to deal with a mixture of complex and simple patient agendas. The pressure of time and short consultation lengths tend to make general practitioners more unwilling to engage with complex patients. A lack of confidence, especially amongst less experienced doctors, can lead to reluctance in engaging with the more difficult problems.

Attendees themselves are acutely aware of time pressures in the GP surgery. Patients with depression have been found to be inhibited from fully disclosing their problems, thus preventing their making best use of the consultation. Doctors should be more aware of patients' anxieties about time and allay these concerns by providing pre-emptive reassurance as a means of reinforcing the attendee's sense of entitlement to consultation time. Patients, particularly those with psychosocial problems, want a patient-centred approach with a doctor who communicates well. Such an approach increases patient satisfaction and leads to fewer investigations being undertaken, and fewer referrals being made.

Patients with psychosocial problems pose quite a challenge, especially when they are presenting for the first time to their doctor who has no previous history or notes to help.

The doctor needs to be particularly canny if the patient has consulted with seemingly physical symptoms, where the underlying problem seems to be psychological; in the majority of cases of these so-called 'medically unexplained symptoms' (MUSs), the psychiatric problem emerges without too much difficulty and without too many unnecessary investigations (see Chapter 1 for further discussion of MUSs).

In the current culture of measurement, targets and quality assurance the unhappy or neurotic person may be presented with a questionnaire to fill in. This is designed to gauge the seriousness of his or her psychological problems. If the matter is clearly related to feelings of unhappiness, the patient can be expected to be questioned about the sensitive subject of suicide (as discussed earlier). And if the scores are high enough on a specific rating scale, this is used to indicate a need for treatment.

The patient-centred approach directs the doctor to adopt a more flexible and consensual stance as compared to the didactic days of old, the aim being to reach an agreement about how to proceed once treatment alternatives have been discussed.

The options include some form of talking treatment, or medication, or simply advice or reassurance or monitoring (sometimes called 'watchful waiting').

Once the patient has been assessed by the GP, the patient might be referred to a psychiatrist or psychologist who has been specifically trained to deal with such conditions. There are many such specialists, and the range is almost bewildering. Patients might see a counsellor, psychologist, psychological wellbeing practitioner (PWP), psychiatrist or a psychotherapist. They may see a community psychiatric nurse (CPN), a social worker or even two or three of the above together. They may see a medical student or a trainee GP if they are in an area where a medical school is located.

The professional the patient first sees after a referral from the GP will usually be part of a team. Here again, the situation can be complicated; the number and types of teams are many, and their names vary between different areas of the country (a full list is given in Chapter 4).

And finally, the actual place where the patient is seen and where the next stage of the process occurs may vary. He or she may continue to be seen in their GP surgery, or the patient may be seen in a larger institution or hospital.

Secondary Care Assessment[33]

The initial stage of specialist psychiatrist or psychologist involvement comprises an in-depth, detailed assessment. This consists of a comprehensive list of questions that follow a general structure, but also allow for some flexibility depending upon what information is gleaned. The aim is to create a better picture of the problem and gauge which direction to proceed in.

For a psychiatrist, the process is really about making a diagnosis. It may be that the patient could then be commenced on some form of medication or that their existing medication may be changed in some way, perhaps by being boosted with an additional drug. Or they may recommend that the patient be seen by another specialist skilled in one of the many varieties of a talking treatment.

The psychologist's assessment overlaps that of the psychiatrist but is also focused on whether or not patients are able to make use of this (psychological) approach, with respect to treatment—in the terms of the trade, 'Are they psychologically minded?' Simply put, this assessment examines if they have the necessary awareness, or the potential to develop the necessary awareness, of psychological processes in order to be helped by such a treatment. Furthermore, the psychologist would seek to establish: 'Do they want to change?' At the end of the assessment process, the decision is made as to whether the sufferer is likely to benefit from talking therapy. Usually some form of feedback interview is conducted and this may also involve discussion of a report written by the assessor. The manner in which the results of the assessment are fed back to the patient may strongly influence their willingness to comply with what is proposed. A brutally realistic report can be as damaging as an unrealistic expectation of cure. A specialist's concluding impressions should be shared with the sufferer with a gentle honesty. Further, the decision not to offer therapy in some circumstances should be carefully explained, so that it is not perceived as a rejection of the individual sufferer. In fact, more often than not it is a reflection of the weakness of current treatments and the system within which they exist.

The usual psychiatric assessment is composed of many discrete subsections, all or some of which may be highly relevant to the difficulties currently faced by the patient (see Chapter 4 for a breakdown of the subsections of the psychiatric assessment).

Sometimes it may be necessary for the health professional to undertake an assessment over several sessions. This should not be seen as a waste of time or an unnecessary delay before treatment can be instituted. For certain neurotic conditions such as adult ADHD and for other problems involving more deep-seated difficulties of the sufferer's character or personality, a longer period of assessment is crucial. It gives the assessor time to get to know the patient and may be invaluable in demonstrating how the symptoms vary from day to day or week to week. Further, it may be necessary for the patient to be assessed using some form of professionally recognised questionnaire, which can be quite lengthy (see Chapter 4 for some examples). Assessment over a number of sessions can allow the doctor the opportunity of getting a corroborative history from a friend or relative. This added interview can be very useful, especially if the collateral story comes from someone who knows the patient well and who has been in contact with them for a long time. For some problems (e.g., personality difficulties) it is especially appropriate to gather additional information about the person from his or her childhood and youth, such as school reports and assessments undertaken by other health professionals, GP records and letters.

It is self-evident that honesty, both on the part of the patient and the assessor, is essential for the assessment process. It may be tempting to embellish or exaggerate one's difficulties, but this can be misleading, and in the long run harmful to the sufferer. Self-diagnosis aided by the internet has pros and cons. On the plus side, some patients who might never have come to the attention of a health professional are motivated to seek help. On the other hand, the cliché 'a little knowledge is a dangerous thing' does often seem to come true. Information gleaned from the internet can frequently be taken out of context of individual variations and complexities of peoples' histories and symptoms. It is easy for most of us to get fixated with a particular issue, and once we become convinced about something it is very difficult to become unconvinced. Disagreeing with the patient who has diagnosed himself or herself often results in complaints, and even legal action against the doctor. *Cyberchondriasis* is the term that has been coined to describe the specific anxiety about illness which has been provoked by information found on the internet.

Forming a clear picture of an individual's problems can be very difficult. For example, psychiatrists are frequently referred patients who have been to see their GP because they think they have bipolar affective disorder or manic depression. Awareness of the illness has increased in recent years particularly after several celebrities including Russell Brand and Stephen Fry revealed they were sufferers.

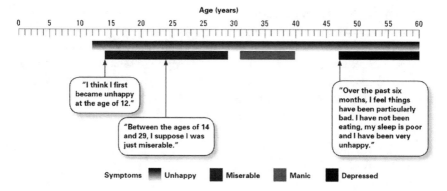

Figure 2. An Example of a Timeline.

To make a diagnosis of manic depression, as has already been stated above, there has to be a pattern of episodes of excessively elevated mood and periods of low mood. Difficulties may arise if the patient has been depressed for a long period of time, and then has a phase of not being low or essentially normal; this phase might be misinterpreted as an episode of elevated mood or mania because the sufferer is so unused to feeling anything other than unhappiness. Such a chronology of events cannot be fully appreciated in a single consultation; careful history taking and interviews with friends and relatives are invaluable here. The use of a mood diary can help to clarify the issues, and the construction of a timeline (as depicted above) may also be informative. The timeline visually depicts patterns of mood variation over time.

Treatments

Introduction

The decision to treat should really only follow a clear diagnosis of disease. Prescribing medication or talking therapies adds weight to the validity of the patient's diagnosis. Recommending treatment further solidifies a diagnosis and *medicalises* it (or in the case of psychological distress, *psychiatrises* it).

The decision to reach for the prescription pad as a solution to a mental illness should never be taken lightly. It is often the case that the drugs are ineffective, or they may worsen the problem, or divert attention away from the root cause of the problems. Drugs may also mask the actual feelings or emotional experiences that are part of the normal spectrum of physiological emotions and reactions. And if these normal human feelings (including anxiety or unhappiness) are to be understood and overcome, then it is necessary for the patient to experience them raw and unfiltered, and not through the prism of pharmacological agents.

Doctors are also cognisant that in many cases patients do not actually take the medication prescribed for them, or may take them in a rather haphazard fashion, on an 'as required' basis. Patients may even take more than they have been prescribed, supplementing them with additional drugs they have purchased over the internet or obtained from friends and relatives. These are commonplace occurrences.

Before the possibility of medication is even considered, other methods and options—if relevant—should be investigated.

Similar caveats apply to the prescription of psychological or talking therapies. These may not always be helpful, and can even be harmful. They may dig up distressing memories. And they may promise the patient false hope of a cure. The alleviation of stress, a change in lifestyle and alternative therapies should be thought about in the management and treatment of neurotic illness, even before the usual mainstream medical options (drugs and/or talking therapies) are adopted.

Lifestyle Considerations

The concept of stress is not a new one. Its role in the causation of mental illness or psychological distress has only become apparent in more recent times. Essentially individuals become stressed when the demands placed upon them become too great to cope with. They become unable to cope with the pressures of life be that at home or at work. Life for most people is not without some degree of stress. It makes us feel unhappy, worried, on edge, apprehensive. It may also produce physical symptoms such as 'butterflies in the stomach', a dry mouth, sweating and a need to go to the toilet.

Some stress (or a degree of healthy anxiety) can be beneficial. It might start the lazy student revising for exams. It might motivate the procrastinating author to finish a piece of work. Such a concept can be represented diagrammatically by the Yerkes Dodson curve, which shows that productivity increases as anxiety (or stress) increases. But too much stress, and productivity drops off. See figure 3.

The symptoms of stress overlap those seen in the neurotic disorders. If the stress becomes severe and pervasive, the sufferer may tip over into a state of depression or anxiety, then needing some form of treatment.

Sleep

A regular amount of sleep is essential for good mental (and physical) health. So too is a normal sleep-wake cycle. Shift work, frequent air travel

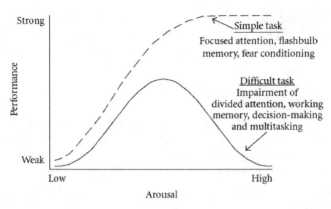

Strong

Weak

Performance

Low   High

Arousal

Simple task
Focused attention, flashbulb
memory, fear conditioning

Difficult task
Impairment of
divided attention, working
memory, decision-making
and multitasking

Figure 3. The Yerkes Dodson Curve Showing Productivity Against Stress.

or simply a lack of routine can upset sleep patterns. This may lead to the development of psychological and psychiatric problems. Irritability, moodiness, grumpiness are common sequelae to insomnia; they are also symptoms of depression, anxiety and other neurotic disorders.

Advice about sleep often given by doctors is labelled, perhaps counter-intuitively, as 'sleep hygiene'. It involves developing a regular pattern, going to bed and waking up at regular times. A number of factors are important: not to drink tea or coffee or other stimulants before bed, being aware that exercise later in the evening may increase alertness and restlessness thereby making sleep more difficult, and gradually winding down in the hours before going to bed. Reading a book or watching television may help us to wind down, but the nature of the material (in books or on the screen) may have the opposite effect—distressing or frightening images may disturb sleep.

Alcohol

Drinking too much alcohol is sometimes the only reason for an individual's unhappiness or anxiety or neurotic symptoms. The logical course of action in such a situation would naturally be to try and cut down, or ideally to try a period of abstinence. In that case, how much should one cut down by, or to? Or how long should one stop drinking for?

To answer these questions, the doctor should consider how much the patient has actually been drinking and his or her patterns of consumption.

Bingeing once or twice a week has been shown to be just as harmful as excessive daily drinking. If patients have actually been drinking for many years, advising them to stop is rather unrealistic; they will probably dismiss such a prescription out of hand and never return. Being pragmatic is more helpful.

Studies have shown that the effects of heavy drinking on brain bio-chemistry and liver function may take weeks or even months to return to normal. Thus, for the patient to expect a miraculous improvement in a matter of days is unrealistic.

Some patients will argue that the consumption of alcohol (or other drugs) does in fact make them feel better. This argument is taken a little further by the patients who declare that they use drugs and alcohol to 'self-medicate'. Some use chemical substances to treat their own psychological or psychiatric problems. Patients typically try a variety of drugs before eventually plumping for a single substance as their 'medication' of choice.

Unsurprisingly, the use of drugs and alcohol to self-medicate is not without problems.

Firstly, continued use (or abuse) of a substance may lead to a degree of dependence. In this situation, it may be that the dependency becomes the main problem and the psychiatric or psychological problem is simply secondary to it.

Secondly, treatments, especially the psychologically based ones such as psychoanalytical psychotherapy, require the patient to be sober and free from withdrawal symptoms in order for the treatment to have an effect on the patient's mental state.

Thirdly, another problem with alcohol (and other drugs) is that they do not combine well with prescription medication. Medication does not get a chance to work if every few days they are washed down with a few glasses of wine or whisky.

Fourthly, patients with an alcohol or drug problem can possess a remarkable capacity for self-deception. Pointing out to the cocaine-snorting financier earning a six-figure salary that it might be worth trying to cut down on the drugs in an attempt to find out if this helps with the problem of anxiety that he or she has been experiencing can often be very difficult. Discussing such an issue needs skill and tact. Further sticking points may arise when he or she requests hypnotic medication to deal with the after effects of the drug, and is denied this because of the pre-existing problems of dependence or addiction.

Finally, the instantaneous effects experienced when, for example, the first vodka shot is swallowed or the first line of coke is snorted is something that the drinker or drug user clearly 'gets off' on. When it is no longer there, he or she will look for something else to replace it. This might be exercise, eating, shopping, or indeed any number of replacement activities. But it is almost certain that the individual does not reach for the medication prescribed by the doctor. Research has shown that the medications prescribed for neurotic disorders do not work immediately. In most cases they do not actually begin to work (or the user will not experience any benefit from them) for at least two, maybe even four weeks. It is also important to bear in mind that they may not work at all—a subject that will be explored further in the next chapter.

Illicit Drugs

The number of illicit drugs available to bring about mind alteration is large. Those currently in vogue include cocaine, MDMA (ecstasy), mephedrone, cannabis (and hydroponic cannabis, skunk), and amphetamines, not to mention all the legal highs such as piperazines, cathinones, phenthylamines, tryptamines and synthetic cannabinoids. They are usually sold as powder and have attractive brand names such as "Spice" or "High Beams". The actual composition of the powder may not always be pure and as with the other more traditional drugs they may be adulterated with a range of different agents.

Prescription drugs are mostly freely available; the internet and globalisation mean that if they cannot be obtained legally in the UK by means of a doctor's prescription, they can easily be purchased elsewhere. Relatives or friends who regularly travel to developing countries can purchase supplies without need for a prescription.

The increasing use of stimulant drinks containing caffeine such as Red Bull is worth bearing in mind as a possible source of mental distress; they may cause anxiety or agitation if consumed in large quantities. They may also cause low mood if not consumed on a regular basis, they may keep the individual awake and thus upset the sleep-wake cycle.

Alternative Therapies

Various over-the-counter remedies are specifically aimed at the treatment of depression or unhappiness. These include St. John's wort and light therapy.

Clear evidence for the effectiveness of St John's wort is lacking. But as it has very few side effects (abdominal pain, sedation and nausea), it is always worth trying if there is a reluctance to take prescribed medication.

Light therapy may likewise be effective in the treatment of unhappiness (more specifically, depression which occurs only in the winter months when there is less natural daylight).[34] Again, the evidence is limited but as with St John's wort there is little harm in trying it out.

If the sufferer is in a state of extremis such that their condition puts their life at risk then popping down to the local health food store for some St. John's wort or purchasing a light box is certainly not recommended.

Physically crippling depression is a medical emergency and should be seen by a GP or hospital doctor immediately.

Food and Exercise

The importance and effectiveness of healthy eating and regular exercise in the treatment of depression still remains equivocal. A highly regarded review combining the results of several studies looking at the effect of exercise on depression concluded that it did seem to improve the symptoms but questions still remain about what type of exercise is most effective. Also, in order for the benefits to be maintained, the exercise probably needs to be maintained in the longer term. This question also needs further research.

With respect to diet, the key ingredient that has received most attention is the omega-3 polyunsaturated fatty acid. The evidence points towards an association of low intake and depression. Such a conclusion comes from studies undertaken in Mediterranean countries where residents consume more vegetables, fruits and nuts, cereals, legumes and fish. Large studies have tended to conclude that such diets are beneficial against depression. There may, of course, be other factors involved.

Generally, it can be appreciated that people with depression may not be able to get themselves together so as to be able to shop for food to make a meal. They may rely on fast food such as burgers and kebabs washed down with fizzy drinks. Such a diet has been shown to have a negative effect upon health, and it can lead to problems with weight and all that entails.

Activity Scheduling

Having daily goals and aims are integral to an individual's feelings of self-worth and value. The need for achievement is universal. In depression and other neurotic illnesses, patients can be helped by setting out in timetables (so-called activity schedules) specific problems that they are avoiding, as well as identifying important tasks they need to undertake. Such activity scheduling begins by getting sufferers to set short-term goals and to regard the timetable as a series of appointments. The most effective results have been achieved by patients starting with small changes in their daily routines and gradually building these up until they are successfully able to carry out more long term aims.

Depressed people tend to avoid activities increasingly as their illness deepens (see figure 4 for examples). The aim should be to focus on those tasks that have been avoided—although in an effort not to make the job too arduous, patients are encouraged to give themselves enjoyable rewards.

> *Social withdrawal*
> a) not answering the telephone
> b) avoiding friends
> *Cognitive avoidance*
> a) not thinking about relationship problems
> b) not making decisions about the future
> *Avoidance by distraction*
> a) watching hours of television
> b) playing computer games
> c) comfort eating
> *Emotional avoidance*
> a) use of alcohol and other substances

Figure 4. Examples of Avoidance in Depression[35].

Summary of Non-Traditional Treatments

It might be somewhat obvious to conclude that the best way to deal with any disease is to stop it developing in the first place. With mental disorders, being aware of how much stress a person can cope with or how much alcohol is being drunk or whether drugs are being taken is an important first step to prevent problems snowballing, and illness developing.

Most employers are aware of the importance of keeping their staff both mentally and physically healthy; this reduces sickness absenteeism, increases morale and improves productivity.

Regular exercise, relaxation classes and other pursuits such as T'ai Chi, meditation, yoga and Pilates are all recommended as helpful activities to improve health and well being.

If the problem is not being defined in medical terms and is thought of as a product of the sufferer's surroundings and society, any remedy found to be helpful can be considered as possible treatment. Friends and family, as well as being important causes of psychological distress, can be important in helping to restore an individual to health. The church or mosque may provide solace to the unhappy or anxious. In a similar way, the local public house may be a source of social interaction and support—providing, of course, that this does not result in the development or encouragement of an alcohol problem.

Medication

Drug treatments for depression, anxiety and the other neurotic disorders are numerous. They are classified into two main groups:

1. Antidepressants
2. Anti-anxiety drugs (known as anxiolytics)

Other drugs may be used, but are usually reserved for more severe cases; these include the antipsychotics and mood stabilisers as well as various 'booster' agents. Finally, electroconvulsive therapy (ECT)—also known as electric shock treatment—may be used, but this is usually a treatment of last resort.

Stephen's Story: Part Six

The endogenous nature of Stephen's illness was striking. The psychologist who had been seeing him for several weeks was convinced that his difficulties clearly appeared to have a biological basis. And, indeed, soon after starting a course of antidepressants, Stephen himself began to notice a change. Firstly, he was less pre-occupied with the hopelessness of his situation although he still continued to mull things over and over in his mind and worry about minute details of how he might organise his life. He still thought he was in a black hole, but gradually he mentioned it less and less. His appetite returned and his sleep improved. And within about three months of starting treatment with an antidepressant Stephen attended his follow-up appointment without a trace of his previously profound unhappiness.

He became a little apprehensive when I said that I felt that his care could continue solely with his GP. But he actually laughed when he hoped he would never see me again. Happily for me (and I hope Stephen) we did meet one more time, but this was by accident in a local park. He was walking along with a woman who he introduced to me as his partner and he told me that he had been thinking about moving out of London. He looked completely different—a confident, cheeky man with a wry smile and a very engaging manner.

Antidepressants

At the latest count there were over 60 different antidepressants listed in the British National Formulary (BNF). There are different classes, but it may be simpler to consider them in two main groups:

1. Selective serotonin reuptake inhibitors (SSRIs), and similar compounds
2. Tricyclic antidepressants (TCAs)

The commoner SSRIs have become household names.[36] Fluoxetine (known by its trade name Prozac) and sertraline (known by its trade names Lustral in the UK, and Zoloft in the United States) are the best examples.

These drugs affect levels of the brain neurotransmitter chemical serotonin. Depression and the other neurotic disorders are thought to be caused by a lack of serotonin and another neurotransmitter called noradrenaline (also known as norepinephrine). The target area for these drugs is known as the synapse (the junction between nerve cells). At the synapse, neurotransmitters are released from one nerve cell, and travel across the gap to reach receptors on the other cell. As part of the cleaning up process after the release of the neurotransmitter, the excess serotonin or noradrenaline is reabsorbed into the original nerve cell, in a process known as reuptake.

There are serotonin and noradrenaline reuptake inhibitors (SNRIs) such as venlafaxine, also noradrenaline and specific serotonin reuptake inhibitors (NaSSAs) like mirtazepine, and noradrenaline reuptake inhibitors (NaRIs) like reboxetine.

The tricyclic antidepressants (TCAs) were one of the first group of drugs developed for the treatment of depression and other neurotic disorders. They act in a similar way to SSRIs by blocking reuptake of serotonin and noradrenaline, but the different TCAs act variably on these two neurotransmitters. They are therefore referred to as 'dirty drugs' because of

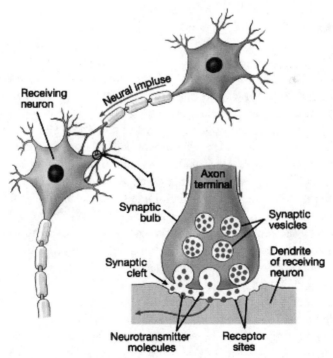

Figure 5. An Annotated Representation of a Synapse and Neuron.

their non-specific mode of action. This characteristic of the TCAs is responsible for their longer list of side effects. Although they are still widely used, they are not recommended as first-line treatment because of the potentially toxic effects they can have on the heart if taken in doses above those recommended. This is really only a problem when there is a risk of suicide with self poisoning or overdose. A full list of TCAs is given in Chapter 4.

Another group, the monoamine oxidase inhibitors (MAOIs), are worth mentioning. Because of their possible serious side effects, they are only prescribed by psychiatrists. They act by boosting levels of neurotransmitters in the brain; but instead of blocking reuptake they prevent them from being broken down. They achieve this by inhibiting an enzyme called monoamine oxidase. The side effect of most importance is the so-called 'cheese and wine reaction'. This unwanted reaction occurs because the MAOIs also stop the breakdown of a constituent of certain foods and drinks, including aged cheese, Chianti wines, Marmite and broad beans. Consumption of such foods while taking an MAOI can lead to interactions which cause a dangerous rise in blood pressure.

There is a recommended treatment protocol for depression that has been developed on the basis of some evidence, and on the experience of specialists prescribing these drugs in practice.

Generally, the first drug prescribed should be an SSRI—and the one found to have the fewest side effects in trials is sertraline. This should be started at the lowest possible dose and if tolerated should be increased in steps up to the maximum recommended dose. At each step increase, the drug should be given time to work—preferably two or three weeks. If, after this time, there has been no change in the level of low mood or anxiety or other symptoms, then it should be increased to the next step. Again, at the higher dose it should be given time to work. This process is repeated until the maximum dose is reached. At the maximum dose, the drug should be trialled for at least two weeks. If, at any step, the individual begins to derive some benefit, that dose should be maintained for at least two to four weeks in order to see if the symptoms are significantly alleviated.

If, after treatment on the maximum recommended dose, there has been no change in the level of depression or other symptoms, then the drug should be gradually decreased. The dose can be reduced every few days and the drug eventually stopped.

What does one do next? Well, if the initial drug was an SSRI, as is usually the case, then it is recommended that a NaSSA or even a NaRI is tried. The next drug can be started at a low dose as the dose of the SSRI is being reduced, to save time (because this can be a lengthy process), and because the risk of interactions is minimal. In essence, both can be prescribed at the same time.

> 1. SSRI – sertraline
> 2. NaSSA – mirtazepine
>   or NaRI – reboxetine
> 3. NaSSA (or NaRI) in
>   combination with TCA

Figure 6. Treatment Protocol for Neurotic Disorders.

The gradual stepwise increase in dose, with regular monitoring for any changes in symptoms, should then be undertaken with the second drug. Again, it should be increased to the maximum if there is no benefit at intermediate doses, and given sufficient time to work.

If, at this stage, drugs from two different classes have failed to alleviate the patient's symptoms, it is still worth trying a different class of antidepressant. This could be a tricyclic (TCA), which can be started while the patient is taking the second drug, but the dose should be low and gradually built up. The aim would be to have the patient taking both drugs at their maximum doses, in combination.

Once the combination of two antidepressants has been tried and failed or partially failed, then it really is time to reassess. If the above treatment protocol has been followed with some diligence, time will have passed, perhaps even a few months, and it may well be that the needs of the sufferer have changed over this time, especially in a first episode of a neurotic disorder. However, if the symptoms of the neurotic disorder are unchanged, careful thought needs to be given to the next step.

At this point, if there has been absolutely no response to the above medication regimes (see figure 6), and it is clear that the sufferer has taken the medication daily as prescribed, then it is worth gradually stopping all and introducing a different one completely.

Venlafaxine, an SNRI is probably the next one to try. This drug has a controversial history, because though it is effective in the treatment of neurotic illness, particularly depression, it has been found to have potential lethal side effects upon the heart. Here again it should be gradually increased in steps, with time taken between dose increments to allow it to work.

If, on the other hand, there were a response to either one or both of the initial medications, it is worth considering boosting or augmenting this effect. Such boosting should be supervised by a specialist because these combinations are not commonly trialled, and because of possible serious side effects. One of the more familiar agents used to boost antidepressants is bupropion (Zyban).[37] Bupropion was originally developed as an antidepressant, but was also found to be effective in helping smoking cessation, and is prescribed more commonly in primary care for this purpose. It is effective on its own but is more commonly used to augment the action of another antidepressant. In combination with an antidepressant that was previously helpful, but has ceased to work alone, buproprion may kick-start the antidepressant effect of the original drug. This combination should be tried for at least four to six weeks.

The other agent commonly used as a booster is lithium.[38] It has many potential side effects such as excessive thirst, excessive urination, metallic taste, weight gain, diarrhoea and constipation. It needs careful monitoring if used for long periods because of the additional side effects of damage to the kidneys and thyroid gland.

Finally, the combination known as triple therapy—of an antidepressant, a booster (usually lithium) and tryptophan—is one of the last resorts.[39]

The drug protocol outlined above may take up to two years to go through. And at that stage if things remain unchanged, there is still room to trial again one of the alternative agents such as duloxetine, agomelatine or mirtazepine. Here again, different combinations with one or other of the different classes can be tried as well as combinations with tryptophan, lithium, or buproprion. Other drugs used in the treatment of neurotic disorders include anticonvulsants, antipsychotics, hypnotics and thyroxine.

Key to this process is that the treating physician should not lose hope. Feelings of desperation on the part of the doctor are quickly transmitted to the patient whose unhappiness may then deepen as a consequence. This can evidently lead to further problems.

Side Effects of Antidepressants

All drugs have possible side effects. The commoner ones attributed to SSRIs and similar antidepressants are:

Nausea
Weight gain or loss
Sexual dysfunction—i.e., an inability to get an erection or an inability to achieve orgasm and a decrease in libido or sexual desire
Nightmares and bad dreams
Dry mouth (particularly the TCAs)
Feelings of anxiousness and panic

It is easy to see that most of these are similar to the symptoms experienced by sufferers with depression, anxiety and other neurotic conditions. As such, it becomes difficult to distinguish whether these are due to the drugs or whether they are part of the neurotic disorder. A common presenting scenario is the unhappy patient who has been prescribed an antidepressant by one doctor, and who consults another, with say, disturbed sleep and requests further medication to rectify the insomnia.

A trial without any antidepressants, especially if the times that various symptoms have developed are unclear, will often resolve both the unhappiness and the side effects.

For a complete list of side effects see Chapter 4.

Withdrawal or Discontinuation Syndrome

Finally, it is necessary to be aware that patients who have taken any antidepressant—but especially the SSRIs—commonly experience a withdrawal syndrome if they stop them. The symptoms are particularly troublesome if the drug has been taken for a few months at a high dose, but can even occur after a few weeks of taking. The way to avoid such a withdrawal (or discontinuation) syndrome is to decrease the drug dose slowly and gradually over a prolonged period.

Common symptoms of the withdrawal syndrome are:

Sleep disturbance and nightmares
Sweating and anxiety symptoms
Mood swings and irritability
Sudden muscle jerks, or feeling an electric shock passing through the head (also known as 'head shocks')

These can be quite unpleasant and continue for a few days or weeks. In exceptional cases they may go on for months. As well as stopping the drug very gradually, it is sometimes recommended that if the individual is on a different SSRI, that this could be changed to fluoxetine (Prozac); the theory is that the withdrawal syndrome with this SSRI is more bearable. This is related to the time taken for the drug to be metabolised by the body, which is longer than the other SSRIs, hence slowing its action (and softening the withdrawal effects).

Serotonin Syndrome

Serotonin syndrome is a potentially fatal reaction that can occur as a consequence of an overdose of serotonergic drugs, or due to drug interactions that increase serotonin levels. There are a range of possible symptoms, from the relatively milder sweating, shivering, and increased heart rate to hyperthermia, agitation and a rise in blood pressure, and even shock, seizures and renal failure. Treatment consists of withdrawing the culprit drug, but sometimes also administering an antidote.

Suicide and the SSRIs

Controversy surrounds the use of SSRIs and an observed increase in suicidal ideas and suicide rates. This first came to light in children who were prescribed the drugs. It was later found to be a problem in adolescents and young adults. However, this has not been causally proven. The Food and Drug Administration in the UK issued several warnings to prescribers to be cautious about the risks involved in treating children and younger adults with these antidepressants. The issue still continues to attract attention and is the subject of repeated analysis. The difficulties lie in the fact that the actual numbers involved are so small, and hence not easy to prove a causal link beyond doubt.

Anti-anxiety Drugs (Known as Anxiolytics)

There are a number of agents targeted at treating anxiety, with variable effects. The most commonly used, by sufferers, is alcohol, which is widely available and used to self-medicate anxiety

Benzodiazepines

Another widely available drug that is very effective in dealing with the symptoms of anxiety is diazepam (known worldwide by its trade name Valium). Diazepam belongs to a class of drugs called benzodiazepines (BDZ). They differ from each other mainly in their duration of action, which translates into the length of time they are able to dampen down the unwanted feelings of anxiety. For example, the effects of temazepam will last only a few hours whereas those of diazepam will last longer.

These drugs are obtained either on prescription from a doctor or illegally with comparative ease, on the street corner (depending upon the quality of one's neighbourhood, of course—although even those in the most salubrious might be surprised about its easy availability).

The benzodiazepines are potent drugs. They do what it says on the packet and they do it well. They do lessen anxiety symptoms and they reduce the stress caused by obsessional thoughts and ruminations. They are successful in overcoming the problems of social phobia, agoraphobia and other specific phobias, and they ease the feelings of unhappiness that are often fuelled by anxiety, and they do all these things within 20 minutes of being consumed.

Unfortunately, such effectiveness comes at a price. This is certainly not financial, as they are very cheap on the street. The price is one of dependence or addiction. They are very addictive drugs and create dependence rapidly. This should not come as a surprise. They get rid of some deeply unpleasant symptoms.

The dependence on benzodiazepines has been said to develop after prolonged use over several weeks, when the person has been taking them more or less daily. In reality, however, they create a powerful pull the moment the sufferer feels the effects for the first time. As soon as anxious or obsessional patients experience an almost instantaneous reduction in their symptoms, they want more of it. They want the effects to carry on and never to stop. There is also the problem of tolerance, in that the individual becomes used to the dose of BDZ, and needs an increase in dose over time to achieve the same effect.

Withdrawal is another significant problem associated with the use of BDZ. Weaning someone off BDZ can be a distressing, lengthy and difficult process. The symptoms of withdrawal are often severe and upsetting. Commonly, the patient will experience:

Anxiety and panic
Tremor
Disturbed sleep
Agitation
Hallucinations and seizures (these symptoms are quite rare)

The process may take weeks or months depending on the length of time that the patient has been taking the drug and the presence of continuing psychological distress or upset in his or her life.

Patients wanting to reduce and come off BDZ should be allowed to do so at their own pace and supported with advice and reassurance. Sometimes it may be necessary in the last stages of the reduction process for the patient to take a fraction of the smallest dose possible for several weeks before they can quit altogether.

The recommendations are, therefore, that these drugs are used with caution, in crises and for a short time only.

The purist and the more psychologically minded may propose that they are never prescribed. They would argue that the drugs are only masking the symptoms; they are simply dampening them down to a tolerable level. The sufferer is not actually dealing with, or facing up to the difficulties, at the root of his or her anxiety symptoms.

In addition, by avoiding the root problems, by masking or covering them up with the drugs, the issues become even more difficult to deal with. Avoidance of a psychological problem means that when the time comes to

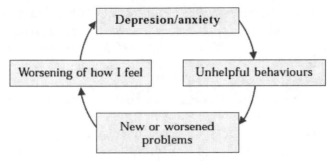

Figure 7. The Vicious Circle of Anxiety and Depression (After Williams et al 2001).[40]
The unhelpful behaviours may be drinking, isolation or taking drugs—anything that stops the sufferer facing up to the problem.

try and deal with it, the anxiety or unhappiness or distress it causes will be even bigger. The individual can get into a vicious circle whereby avoidance leads to increasing difficulty in facing up to the problems, which leads to further avoidance, which leads to even more difficulty facing up to the problem and so on.

The biologically orientated doctor may willingly prescribe benzodiazepines. And they may be effective in some cases. If the sufferer is going through a crisis such as a bereavement or breakdown in family relationships, then a short course of diazepam may enable them to navigate and survive the calamitous situation they find themselves in.

They may be prescribed during an episode of depression and anxiety alongside an antidepressant, just to help the sufferer through the early days before the antidepressant 'starts to kick in'.[41]

The more psychologically orientated doctor may do nothing other than recommend that the patient see a counsellor or psychologist as soon as possible. Alternatively, the doctor may take a little extra time out of his or her busy surgery and talk through the difficulties with the patient presenting in crisis.

If there is an element of suicidal risk in the patient's presentation, the appropriate action may be immediate referral for psychiatric assessment, and possibly hospital admission, or possibly crisis psychotherapeutic intervention. However, as often happens, the problem may simply resolve spontaneously and the more conservative listening (rather than biological) approach may be the best tactic. And the risk of dependence on benzodiazepines is avoided.

Unfortunately, there are many patients who are now dependent on BDZ, having first been prescribed them several years ago, perhaps when the risks and dangers were not so well recognised. They were not weaned off BDZ soon enough, with dependence developing swiftly, and making individuals extremely reluctant to come off these drugs. This has become a difficult issue for a significant minority of patients, with many blaming their doctors for prescribing these drugs in the first place. Often a present-day doctor is left to answer for a colleague who is long gone and has to address the pragmatic issue of how (or even if) to wean someone off these highly addictive drugs, after many years of consumption.

Hypnotics

Sleep disturbance is one of the commonest reasons for patients consulting their doctor. If practical strategies and sleep hygiene have not worked, short courses of hypnotics may be prescribed.

The BDZ are prescribed as hypnotics. Zopiclone and the other so-called z drugs, zolpidem and zaleplon, are non-benzodiazepine hypnotics, which have some overlap (with BDZ) in the way they work. Zopiclone is particularly effective as a short-term solution for insomnia and it has few troublesome side effects; it might cause the patient to feel a bit groggy or 'hung over' the morning after its consumption.

The z drugs were initially thought to not have the problems of dependence, tolerance and withdrawal which BDZ do, and were marketed as such. However, time has shown that these significant side effects similarly occur with the z drugs, and they are no safer than BDZ.

Melatonin is also used in insomnia or sleep disturbance. It is a naturally occurring hormone, which is important in the sleep-wake cycle. It has been used for jet lag and other short-term sleep disturbances.

Tryptophan

Tryptophan is an essential amino acid that cannot be synthesised in the human body, and needs to be ingested. It is found in most protein-based foods, including milk, eggs, fish, poultry, oats, chocolate and sunflower/ pumpkin seeds. Tryptophan is used in the synthesis of both serotonin and melatonin in the body, and has been trialled in low serotonin conditions such as depression. It has been shown to be effective particularly when used to augment the action of another antidepressant. However, the jury is still out on the extent of its efficacy.

Thyroxine

Thyroxine is a naturally occurring hormone produced by the thyroid gland. Both increased and decreased levels of thyroxine are associated with features of anxiety and depression. Limited trials have shown that it could be combined with an antidepressant in patients who have only had a partial response to the latter.

Sodium Valproate and Other Related Anticonvulsants

Drugs used by neurologists in the treatment of epilepsy have also been used by psychiatrists in the treatment of various mood disorders including bipolar affective disorder, cyclothymia[42] and dysthymia.[43] They work by dampening down fluctuations in mood, and by preventing the development of troublesome highs and lows. They are a last resort for sufferers with mild to moderate mood disturbances. They may have an active effect upon decreasing the mood in patients who are 'high', but their main use is to prevent the actual ups and downs developing in the first place. They have a long list of potential side effects some of which may be life threatening. Most patients on these drugs need regular monitoring and medical supervision, including blood tests.

Pregabalin is an antiepileptic drug that has been licensed for use in the treatment of anxiety disorders as a second or third-line drug. It is also used to treat neuropathic and chronic pain. It seems to have much less potential for addiction and abuse than the benzodiazepines, but is also far more expensive than many first line drugs. It may also be used in combination with an antidepressant.

Antipsychotics

In some cases, the feelings of despair or anxiety or other neurotic symptoms can become so severe and totally overwhelming that the sufferer loses touch with reality. They may develop strong beliefs of hopelessness or persecution such that they fear that others are trying to harm or kill them. They may come to believe that the only way out of their misery is to commit suicide. They may reach a state where they actually believe they are in fact dead, or that various parts of their body are rotting away or dead. If their distress reaches this profound level, they may be diagnosed as being psychotic, leading to consideration of treatment with an antipsychotic.

These drugs should not be used lightly. They have many side effects, some of which can be irreversible, especially amongst the older drug families, though even the modern antipsychotics are also not trouble free.

Antipsychotic drugs can be classified in a variety of ways which have been much debated, but still fall into the two easy, broad categories of 'old' and 'new'. The best-known and most widely used 'old' antipsychotic is chlorpromazine, which was first produced in the 1960s. The newer drugs include risperidone, olanzapine, and quetiapine. It is of note that many of the newer drugs have also been found to have an antidepressant effect and have also been used either in combination with one of the SSRIs or tricyclics.

Margaret's Story

Unhappiness can often be seen in the facial expressions of sufferers and Margaret was no exception. She had a furrowed brow with lines so deep and so contorted that they provided a clear indication of the depth of the emotional turmoil she was feeling on the inside. She was in her early 60s and had been under my care for more than three years before things suddenly changed. I have to say that I had almost given up hope of any improvement when, in the course of my adopted protocol for treating patients with depression, we had almost reached the end of the road together. She was taking two antidepressants from two different classes, an antipsychotic and the latest drug I decided to add, which was lithium. The change was remarkable. After two months of a reasonably low dose, the furrows had gone completely. So noticeable was the smoothness of her forehead, that I barely recognised her as she skipped down the corridor from the waiting area to my consulting room. Previously it had been like a grey cloud descending, now she was like a ray of sunshine. I could not believe it.

Margaret herself said she could not believe the change either. She had stopped smoking, she had begun to socialise again and specifically said that she had been able to taste her food for the first time in nearly five years.

She said that she did not know how to thank me. I explained that just to see her without her furrowed brow had made my afternoon. She laughed, shook my hand and said she hoped she would never see me again!

Electroconvulsive Therapy (ECT)

Electroconvulsive therapy (ECT) has gained an unjustified reputation as being the quintessential treatment approach of psychiatrists towards the mentally ill. It is used only as a last resort in the treatment of profoundly ill depressed or manic patients. In depression, it should be seen as the treatment to try when all other combinations of antidepressants have failed, and there exists an emergency situation in which the patient has reached a state of wretchedness so extreme that they have virtually shut down mentally and physically. They are not eating, they are losing weight, they are moving slowly and have simply lost the will to live, with a frailty that points to an almost inevitable outcome of death, unless there is a radical external intervention.

When used appropriately, in severe treatment-resistant cases, ECT has been shown to be effective. However, it does not seem to have sustained benefit, and individuals often need subsequent treatment with other modalities.

It is administered to an anaesthetised patient who is asleep in the form of an electric shock, which is applied using electrodes placed on one or both sides of the head. This produces a controlled epileptic-like seizure lasting several seconds. It is unclear how this form of treatment can cause a change in mood. ECT can cause significant memory loss, a frightening side effect that most are aware of.

Stimulants and Treatments for ADHD

The idea of using a stimulant drug to help an individual whose problems involve inattention, increased activity and impulsivity may seem rather counterintuitive, but the mainstay of treatment for patients with attention deficit hyperactivity disorder are drugs related to amphetamines (also known as 'speed').

The theme of using any drug to enhance performance or improve lifestyle, which is what happens with the successful treatment of ADHD, is one that continues to generate much controversy. Healthcare professionals and academics tend to adopt rather polarised views in opposing camps.

The psychiatrist needs to make the difficult judgement about whether the sufferer's symptoms fall well outside the normal range of experience. This distinction is even more crucial in ADHD—particularly in adult cases—because the treatments can lead to positive results even in the 'normal' person. To reiterate the point, the medications will help some people to perform better; they may concentrate for longer, they may be able to stay up later at night studying or they may just feel more alert even if they do not have ADHD. This is a fairly unique feature of the amphetamine drugs used in the treatment of this condition. Drugs such as antidepressants do not have a positive effect upon the mood of a normal individual. This should make the prescriber of stimulant drugs very wary.

Issues concerning ADHD in children are somewhat different. Child and adolescent psychiatrists are generally very cautious about prescribing stimulant medications to their patients, taking into account several hours of observation of the child in a variety of settings (including school and the family home) as well as interviewing a number of professionals involved with the child (such as teachers and social workers) before they conclude that drug treatment is the right option.

In adults, the state of affairs is often more complicated for a number of reasons.

Firstly, many of the adult patients presenting to their GP or local psychiatrist have not been diagnosed locally, and detailed assessment notes and letters are lacking. Reappraisal of the diagnostic process is always important, especially in a condition that is so contentious, and where professional and societal attitudes vary from country to country. By the same token, assessment and diagnosis in another country presents even more obstacles in re-examining the authenticity and rigour of diagnosis.

Secondly, the sufferer may not have been assessed as a child and may be presenting for the first time with complaints about attention and concentration, which must be differentiated from other psychiatric or psychological problems including depression, anxiety and other neurotic conditions.

Thirdly, the sufferer has often researched their problems and become convinced of the diagnosis, therefore being keen to start medication as soon as possible. They have often completed various validated questionnaires online, which have simplistically concluded with a diagnosis of ADHD, and directed them to seek a prescription from a doctor. (See chapter 3 for a sample of one commonly used screening tool for adults.)

The NICE guidelines recommend drugs as the first line of treatment in patients with a clear diagnosis of ADHD. However, in practice, approaches to treatment are more measured and there is no universal rush to prescribe stimulant medication as a first line for all patients.

When drug treatment is deemed to be important, most doctors try methylphenidate in the first instance. The medication comes in two forms: modified (or slow release) and unmodified (or immediate release). The latter is popularly known by its trade name, Ritalin, and is usually taken three or four times a day. The drug takes about 40 minutes to work and its effects last for at least two hours.

The modified form is a combination of the immediate release medication and the sustained release, thus enabling the patient to take just one dose daily.

The side effects of methylphenidate are similar to most stimulants and include anxiety and feelings of being on edge, tremor, irritability, insomnia and disturbed sleep, weight loss and appetite suppression, and occasionally even the development of psychotic symptoms such as delusions or hallucinations. Stimulant medications also have potentially serious effects on the cardiovascular system, such as cardiac rhythm abnormalities and significant rises or lowering in blood pressure. Cardiac monitoring and blood tests are therefore needed prior to starting these drugs, and at intervals while the individual continues to take them.

The second line drug of choice after methylphenidate is atomoxetine. It is apparently not as stimulating as methylphenidate but also runs the risk of cardiovascular problems as well as sexual dysfunction including decreased libido and urinary retention.

The third line is an amphetamine. In the UK this drug is only available on the NHS in the 'dextro' form, i.e., dexamphetamine or dextroamphetamine. The 'dextro' prefix simply indicates that it is the right-hand isomer of the drug; the other form is the left-hand 'levo' isomer.[44] In the USA and on private prescription in the UK, psychiatrists commonly prescribe a combination of both isomers better known by its trade name Adderall. There is a generally held belief that the drug in combination form is more stimulating than the dextro form on its own, a possible explanation for the observation that patients visiting the UK from abroad seem dissatisfied with a prescription for their medication in the British dextro form.

Finally, it is also worth remembering, and pointing out to patients desperate to start treatment, that, even with stimulant drugs, there is a well recognised placebo effect, which in some trials has been shown to manifest in up to 30% of patients. This means that even amongst sufferers of ADHD, about one third will feel better when treated with a dummy tablet that contains no active ingredients.

Talking Treatments

The rise in the popularity of talking cures or psychological therapies as alternatives to medications in the treatment of depression and other neurotic conditions has been meteoric. In the last five years the use of psychotherapy treatments has expanded still further, with the development of a service aimed at speeding up and improving access for all sufferers.

However, methods of curing unhappiness and other forms of mental illness or distress by talking are probably as ancient as conversation itself. A mother counselling her worried daughter or a father encouraging his unconfident son or friends reassuring each other has happened throughout history. Today modern ideas about psychological therapies are well established and supported by a raft of clinical trials and research. Yet even though there are several different approaches to the ways therapists currently deliver treatments using a variety of methods or frameworks, the most important aspect to the whole process is the so-called therapeutic relationship or alliance. Essentially this is how the therapist and the patient interact; it is the component common to all types of talking treatment and it is fundamental to the therapy being successful.

Patients usually see their therapist on a weekly basis, although this may vary and in some cases sessions may take place every two or three days for several years. Such a service is rarely available on the NHS and the more usual practice is for the therapist to see his or her patient (or client) once a week for about 16 sessions. There may be an assessment session before the actual therapy starts and there is usually a final debriefing once the treatment has been completed; the therapist may give the patient a summary of his or her findings along with a formulation of the problems.[45]

In 2006, in a backlash against the increasing use of antidepressants and the alleged medicalisation of societal distress, plans to expand access to psychological therapies were unveiled by economics guru Professor Lord Richard Layard. The project involved the training of some 10,000 therapists over a seven-year period who would be easily accessible in general practices and job centres. Lord Layard relied upon the NICE guidelines for authority when he called for most patients with depression and anxiety disorders to be offered psychological treatment. It may be unfair to say that money was the main motivator for the Government to implement the plan with so little evidence for its effectiveness, but according to Layard: 'such treatments yield economic benefits that exceed the cost'. He added: 'There is no net cost to the Government because of savings on incapacity benefits and other NHS costs'.[46]

The attractiveness of this proposal could not be ignored, especially in the context of recent concerns about the effectiveness of drug treatments for neurotic illnesses and long waiting lists for psychological therapy—in most cases up to six months.

However, as with the initial beliefs about the effectiveness of medication, claims about the benefits of psychological treatments were probably over estimated. And the alleged reductions in numbers of claimants of various benefits will probably never materialise.

Counselling

Counselling is a broad term used in mental health services to mean any type of therapeutic psychotherapy. However, the purists would generally take it to refer to a form of talking therapy that is short in duration, orientated specifically towards helping patients use their own resources to resolve problems of a less severe nature. The following two organisations are given by way of examples of counselling services widely available. They are both national organisations and one (MIND) has local branches throughout the UK. Other counselling services are available for specific problems in certain parts of the country.

1. **MIND**
   The organisation provides many different services including crisis helplines, drop-in centres, counselling, befriending, advocacy, employment and training schemes.
   http://www.mind.org.uk/

2. SANE

SANE provides supportive counselling over the phone or via its new email service SANEmail.
http://www.sane.org.uk/

Cognitive Behavioural Therapy

Cognitive behavioural therapy (CBT) is one of the best-researched and fastest-growing types of psychological therapy. There is a great deal of research supporting its effectiveness and it is recommended by the NICE guidelines as the treatment of choice for many psychological conditions including depression, anxiety, agoraphobia, obsessive compulsive disorder and ADHD. As a general rule of thumb, CBT is thought to be most effective when the problem has reached a moderate to severe level; for more mild conditions results are less impressive.

The CBT model is based on the concept that cognitions (i.e., thoughts), feelings, behaviours and biological factors are interlinked in the presentation of a psychological problem. The therapist aims to work with sufferers to help them change their negative thoughts and unhelpful behaviour patterns. For example, a patient (or client in the psychologist's parlance) with depression should learn to identify his or her negative thoughts and try to gain more of a balanced perspective of them.

A sufferer of agoraphobia will need to learn to manage his or her anxiety symptoms through gradual exposure to the source of the worry: commonly crowded places. The treatment might involve going to busier and busier places every day or week, for example. Concomitantly, during the process of building up to more and more crowed areas, the patient will be asked to keep testing out the thoughts and ideas that originally caused the fear.

One of the main advantages of CBT is that it can be a relatively short treatment with good results. Depending on the severity of the problem, the sufferer will need between eight and 20 sessions lasting 50 minutes each. It can be delivered on an individual basis and also in groups, focusing on more on so-called psycho education, during which time the therapist basically teaches the clients about their problem from a psychological perspective and introduces them to the CBT type skills. Most CBT therapists hold qualifications as psychologists, counsellors or psychotherapists or they may be professionals from other disciplines, such as nurses and occupational therapists, who have completed a specialist CBT training. There are recognised CBT training programmes throughout the UK that are regulated by the British Association for Behavioural and Cognitive Psychotherapies (BABCP).

Many other therapies share common theoretical ground with CBT. These have been developed as treatments for specific psychological conditions or with a focus on particular therapeutic aspects of CBT. These are sometimes referred to as 'Third Wave' cognitive and behavioural therapies or are seen as standalone treatments. Some of the most popular and those most likely to be available on the NHS are briefly described below. For most of these therapeutic treatments there are no specific regulatory bodies so it is recommended that therapists using them should be recognised by a relevant awarding or professional body including the BABCP, the British Psychological Society (BPS) or United Kingdom Council for Psychotherapy (UKCP). In addition, most therapists working in the NHS also need to be recognised by the Health and Care Professions Council (HCPC).

1. Mindfulness Based Cognitive Therapy (MBCT)
Mindfulness is described as a state of focusing complete attention from moment to moment on one's present experiences. It has its origins in Eastern philosophies and meditation practices. It was adapted as a therapeutic approach specifically by CBT practitioners who recognized its potential to extend their skills within the framework of their original model.

Mindfulness-based cognitive therapy specifically helps clients identify, challenge and change their thoughts. The hope is that once the patient has observed these thoughts and identified them as being important in the way they feel, they can then let them go.

Through mindfulness skills development and practice, both in and outside the session, clients learn to redirect their attention away from those thoughts that are causing distress to other parts of their experience in the present, such as their breathing or specific sounds or other senses triggered by their environment.

Currently there is insufficient evidence to support the superiority of this approach over others but a recent rise in interest and research in this method may soon provide empirical data to support its widespread use in the future.

2. Acceptance and Commitment Therapy (ACT)
Acceptance and commitment therapy shares some of the principles found in mindfulness practice and philosophy. It helps the client identify their thoughts, understand how they affect them emotionally and accept them. It is based on the principle that struggling against unwanted thoughts is like struggling in quicksand: it only makes you sink deeper. In sessions, therapists aim to help patients learn to accept their state of mind and as a consequence 'float' and improve their experiences. The hope is that clients learn to develop a new perspective on their experiences; they aim to

identify those values that are most important in their lives and then draw up a plan that will help enable them to be adopted.

3. Compassion Focused Therapy (CFT)

Compassionate focused therapy has been described as a transtheoretical approach, which really means that it integrates and uses elements of several different psychological theories and approaches. It was initially developed through work with people with severe and chronic depression. For it was observed that people with such problems were highly self-critical and prone to experiencing shame. They also shared common themes in their early life experiences, such as being cared for by their mother or father who showed them little warmth or affection.

As part of the package of care, CFT offers psychoeducation to the clients helping them specifically to understand how the brain responds to perceived threats and how its different parts play different roles in regulating emotions.

In addition, patients are meant to learn to identify key fears or threats triggered in different situations along with the protective strategies that might be employed to deal with such experiences. The hope is that through a variety of explicit techniques and the therapist's guidance, clients learn to be more self-compassionate or understanding towards their own feelings.

The CFT approach is very much based on the principle that change cannot be reached purely on a cognitive level but needs to be experienced on an emotional level through the activation of the self-soothing part of the brain. More specifically, a person who has never experienced themselves as lovable may struggle to challenge negative views about themselves. They may conclude, for example, that: 'I am unlovable'. The therapy's aim is to strengthen the part of the brain responsible for positive feelings about themselves and hopefully make the sufferer experience themselves as lovable.

4. Schema Therapy

Schema therapy originates in the concept of a schema, which is defined by psychologists as the internal structure that helps everyone to understand and interpret information. Schema therapy is based on the notion that such structures stem from the person's past experiences. They inform the way we view ourselves, others and the world. The aim of schema therapy is to help the person identify their own interpersonal patterns and coping behaviours, and then to update and modify them.

Schema therapy integrates several ideas from psychology including those of CBT, attachment theory, and psychodynamic psychotherapy (see below).[47] Through the use of a variety of different techniques, such as imagery, along with the actual therapeutic relationship, clients are allowed to experience different aspects of themselves in an attempt to change unhelpful behavioural patterns. Schema therapy offers patients an elaborate description of the patterns of their relationships and aspects of their personality, which are referred to as 'schema modes and domains'. The actual therapy may usually last more than a year and has been shown to be effective with more treatment-resistant problems such as intractable depression and deep seated personality issues.

5. Cognitive Analytic Therapy (CAT)
As its name implies, cognitive analytic therapy combines the elements of both cognitive therapy and psychoanalytic theory. It involves the therapist using the same interactive treatment style of CBT but it is also informed by a more psychoanalytical understanding the client's interpersonal style (see below for a more detailed explanation of psychoanalysis). Patient and therapist work in collaboration to produce a formulation of the problem that aims to pull together all parts of the sufferer's past experiences and the current difficulties. In therapy, the client will explore how early experiences form so-called reciprocal roles (RRs) in his or her relationships. For example, if the client grew up in an abusive environment where the resultant feelings were those of worthlessness, then it is likely he or she would perceive other relationships in adult life in a similar. The final outcome might be that such patients would feel and behave in a similar way to when they were a child.

Through a process of formulation, reformulation and revision at different stages of therapy, clients gain an understanding of the negative vicious cycles that maintain their problems. They also learn 'exit' strategies that help them out of those cycles. One characteristic element of this type of therapy is the exchange of letters between client and therapist. The therapist shares a written formulation with the client in the middle stages of therapy, which they update together. At the end of therapy they both write to each other summarising what the patient has learned and achieved during their work together. There is not enough empirical evidence to recommend CAT over other treatments, but some studies suggest it is most effective in patients with eating disorders and more deep-seated personality difficulties. One advantages of this type of therapy is that it can be relatively short in duration, ranging between eight and 24 sessions.

6. Dialectical Behavioural Therapy (DBT)
The term *dialectical* refers to the process of examining two opposing concepts and finding the balance between them. In DBT this process takes place between change and acceptance, two of the main skills employed as

part of the therapy. These two concepts appear conflicting but the aim is for the clients to be able to incorporate them both in their lives. Clients learn to accept, for example, their past and the things they have no control over, but also to change what they can control, like their behaviour.

Dialectical behavioural therapy is another type of therapy that integrates elements of different approaches such as mindfulness, CBT, and psychodynamic theory. It is a skills based therapeutic program where patients usually take part in both group and individual sessions. They are explicitly taught skills in the group, such as the tolerance of distress, emotion regulation and mindfulness (see above). And during individual therapy sessions they are supported through the application of these skills to real life situations. It is usually a long-term treatment and can last over a year. Therapists sometimes provide more general type of support to patients in treatment as well, which can result in them being available to them out-of-hours. This extensive support is mainly offered to clients at high risk of suicide, self-harm and those with deep seated personality difficulties.

Psychodynamic Psychotherapy

Psychodynamic therapy has its roots in the earliest forms of talking therapy, psychoanalysis, which was conceived by the 'father' of psychology, Sigmund Freud. The aim is for the patients to gain insights into the so-called unconscious forces that both lead to their distress and guide their behaviours. The therapy's main focus is usually on the client's past and the types of attachments they made during childhood.

The therapist aims to understand how such early experiences impact on the patient's adult interpersonal style and the client's experience of unwanted feelings. The relationship between therapist and client is particularly important in this approach. Therapists use their observations of how the client relates to them during therapy (transference) but also their own emotional reactions towards the patient (counter transference). Both transference and counter transference are used to make interpretations of these observations. The therapist's stance is usually less directive or interactive than in other types of therapy. And the actual course of treatment may last many months continuing on in extreme cases for several years. Psychodynamic psychotherapy can be given individually, in groups, to couples and to families. Its theory and practice has evolved over the years and there are now many different schools with a variety of different approaches to this type of therapy.

Although it is one of the oldest psychological treatments, research evidence for its efficacy has been relatively limited, partly due to the nature of this treatment such that it is based on interpretation rather than empirical testing. In recent years research into this type of treatment has yielded positive outcomes when specifically used to treat chronic and complex mental disorders.

As described above, psychodynamic theory has been integrated with cognitive and behavioural therapies in the development of new approaches (such as CAT). There are, however, a number of other therapies currently used in the NHS where a psychodynamic-type approach has been developed to treat specific mental health problems. Two of these are described below.

1. *Mentalisation Based Treatment (MBT)*

Mentalisation has been defined as a one's capacity to understand the mental processes (for example intentions, beliefs and needs) that guide one's behaviour. The aim of therapy is for patients to develop their so-called mentalisation capacity in order that they might gain insight into their own and others' behaviours. Through this process, it is hoped that clients might become more in control of both their emotional reactions and their behaviours. Informed by psychodynamic theory, MBT focuses on offering a secure attachment base from where the client can safely reflect and test out their understanding of 'the mind of the other'. This type of therapy has been tailored around the needs of clients with deep-seated personality difficulties. It has a reasonable body of evidence supporting its effectiveness and is usually only available at more specialist centres in the NHS. It is usually provided as part of a more extensive MBT program involving both group and individual therapy. It may last over a year.

2. *Interpersonal Psychotherapy (IPT)*

This type of therapy is also informed by psychodynamic theory as its focus is mainly on how interpersonal factors affect a person's experience of distress. However, it is not always seen as a psychodynamic approach as it is shorter in duration continuing for between 12 and 16 sessions. It is problem focused and has a more directive nature; clients work with specific goals and learn techniques that can help them manage their difficulties. It is tailored to helping people diagnosed with depression but has also been shown to be effective with patient with a wide range of problems including bipolar disorder and bulimia nervosa.

Family and Couples Therapy

As the name suggests, family therapy is an approach that involves the client's family in the course of treatment. The 'family', which may include relatives, spouses or any other significant people in the client's life, attend sessions together with the client. Therapists (there are usually more than one involved in the sessions) interact with the family, observe and then reflect upon the interactions between them. The focus of therapy is to understand the client's psychological problems within the context of their interactions with other family members, rather than focusing on the processes within the individual.

Therapists observe the role each family member takes on and how these are related to the way they experience and communicate their needs and feelings to each other. There are many different strands of family therapy originating in different theories, such as psychodynamic and systemic, but an overall aim of this approach is to improve the communication between family members and to help them find better ways of managing distress.

Family therapy has been shown to be effective in patients suffering with a wide range of psychological problems including schizophrenia, bipolar disorder, eating disorders and alcohol dependence.

Conclusion

'The drugs don't work, they just make you worse . . .'—a memorable line from a pop song by the Verve is a pithy reminder of needing to adopt a cautious approach to the drug treatment of mental illness. The drugs used in psychiatry, and particularly in the more poorly defined nebulous neurotic illnesses, work imperfectly, run the risk of side effects and are often unpredictable on an individual basis. The drugs, especially the antidepressants, have been subjected to research trials, with varying degrees of rigour and analysis. In randomised controlled trials (RCTs) and meta-analyses, the antidepressants have mostly been shown to be superior to placebo.

In 2008, however, a shocking study was published, seeming to show that SSRIs were no better than placebo in the treatment of depression.[48] The scientific analysis was systematic and rigorous, and the researchers had obtained data on all the clinical trials submitted to the U.S. Food and Drug Administration (FDA). This information had not been made available fully in the past, and had not been included to its full extent in previous analyses of the data. It seemed to point towards a conspiracy by pharmaceutical companies who it was alleged were being selective with data to make their products appear more effective than they actually were. Much debate ensued. And the matter, understandably, still continues to provoke much argument in the scientific literature.

The truth is probably somewhere in between. Antidepressants may not be as effective as they were once thought to be, except in moderate to severe depression.

Most practitioners of psychological talking treatments are convinced about their effectiveness in the treatment of mental health difficulties. Difficulties arise with proving that they work and more complex still is trying to understand how they work. Most studies have been done with psychologists using CBT on patients with a narrow range of disorders including depression, anxiety and phobias. Additionally, the focus has been on patients with moderate to severe problems, rather than the more prevalent range of mild problems.

On the whole, when compared with placebo, psychological therapy has been shown to be effective. However, one large study did conclude that talking therapies in many cases were no better than placebo.[49] Psychologists responded to this criticism well, and talking therapies for mental illness continue to expand. But, they are not without limitations. For more long-term difficulties, a short course of CBT is ineffective and may even make things worse by stirring up hidden, long-repressed emotions and feelings. And by virtue of simply attending and expecting change, patients may feel let down and disappointed at the end of the treatment course when they finds that their problems remain unchanged. Unhappiness and anxiety that have been developing since childhood require longer-term psychotherapy, which may not be available on the NHS, because of the time and cost-intensive nature of this therapy. If the individual decides to seek help privately, this may mean significant cost over many years.

At the heart of the success of talking therapies is simply the relationship that develops between the patient and the therapist. The relationship is key to the therapeutic nature of the therapy. This is as important with lay counsellors offering support in the voluntary sector as it is with the _über_ qualified medical consultant psychotherapist. The therapy is unlikely to work without a good patient-therapist relationship.

The clinical judgement of a doctor is still crucial in deciding what treatments are offered, and will vary from individual to individual. They cannot be prescribed in formulaic manner for the subtle, complex, ever-varying presentations of mental illness, despite the stipulations of NICE guidelines. NICE guidelines are useful only as a general approach or checklist to ensure that all aspects have been considered.

Generally, a doctor should seek a better understanding of the problem by going to the trouble of exploring the issues further, before suggesting treatment. This takes time, but is a wiser strategy, unless there is any significant risk involved, either to the patient harming themselves or others.

Risk of harm to self or others may need quick action, including inpatient admission.

Regarding a decision about drug treatment or psychological therapy, it must be remembered that neither will bring about instantaneous results. The best course of action may be to do nothing. It may well be that the problem will resolve on its own, and simply explaining the situation and the resulting symptoms the individual is experiencing, and reassurance about this will suffice.

CHAPTER 3

Outcomes

Introduction

An understanding of the course and outcome of an illness offers patients, health care professionals and carers alike invaluable insight into what they might expect to face in the future. This is particularly true in cases of mental illness where stigma and the often distressing nature of the conditions encountered might frighten loved ones away. The patient might then become isolated and feel even more rejected by friends and family.

Such isolation is often more keenly felt in patients with depression, anxiety and the other neurotic conditions. The reason for this is twofold. Firstly, sufferers remain very much aware of their surroundings; they are not so ill that they lose touch with reality. They therefore are usually fully cognisant of any negative attitudes directed towards them. Secondly, because they display symptoms that are essentially an extension of the normal human experience they tend to be thought of as less impaired or less ill. And those who come into contact with them might then believe that they should simply 'pull themselves together'.

The First Episode Outcome

A good starting point in considerations of the outcomes of neurotic illness is to appreciate whether the sufferer has had difficulties before. The past having an important bearing upon future outcome. In patients presenting for the first time, i.e., without ever having had problems before, the outcome is different from those with recurrent illness. However, in reality, such a distinction is problematic. No one has a completely clean slate of past experiences. Everyone has had an episode of unhappiness or a touch of anxiety, for example, before they seek help from a health care professional.

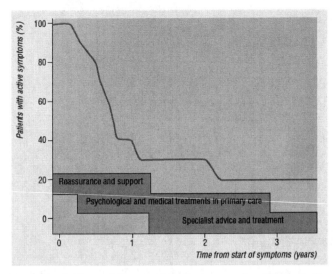

Figure 8. The Resolution of Depressive Symptoms in All New Cases (Craig 1995).

Therefore, it is easier to look at the outcomes of people presenting for the first time to their doctor with symptoms of depression or anxiety or any other neurotic illness.

In the majority of cases the feelings will go away in a matter of weeks. This is true whether they are receiving some form of treatment or not.

Looking at figure 8, it can be seen that the number of patients with active symptoms plummets from 100 to about 40 in the first few months and by the end of the first year about 75% of people are well. Following the line further along, it can be seen that by the end of the second year 80% of patients no longer have problems.

The same excellent improvement rate is seen in patients with so called medically unexplained symptoms. About 70% resolve spontaneously within a few months. In patients with PTSD, the outcome in the first 12 months is also extremely good with up to 80% resolving.

Interestingly enough, the number of people taking time off sick follows the same rapidly resolving prognosis, although here it is even better. Looking at 100 people attending their GP for a sick certificate for the first time, it has been found that up to 95 of them will be back to work within the year.[50]

Finally, computer generated predictions of outcomes of patients with first episodes of depression have produced very similar results (see figure 9).

In summary, most people with neurotic disorders improve rapidly within the first few weeks if they are new cases. In addition, it has been found that the same excellent outcome is seen in both patients with

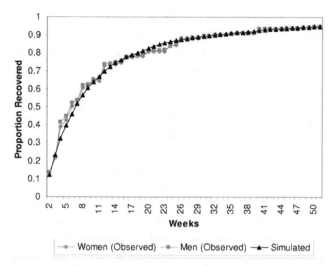

Figure 9. Observed and Simulated Episode Duration Data, by Sex (Patten 2005).[51]
The outcomes are shown as the increasing proportion recovered over time.

symptoms indicating just one disorder, e.g., depression, and in patients with multiple symptoms indicating a more mixed picture of illness. To reiterate this point, it does not seem to matter if the patient has just two symptoms of depression (for example, a low mood and tiredness) or whether they have many symptoms of several neurotic disorders (for example, features of anxiety, obsessional ruminations, unhappiness, and a fear of going out in crowds). Either way, the outcome is the same. The situation is reinforced by research that has found that even when patients were ill enough to merit input from secondary care psychiatric services, two out of five are still improved within a few weeks.

An understanding of such positive outcomes is found in the way we commonly deal with our problems. People tend to go to seek help in times of crises. Essentially they just cannot 'take anymore'. In the majority of cases bringing the issues out in the open so to speak enables them to be sorted out, or at the very least they can begin to be sorted out.

Outcomes after Repeated Episodes

When the person has been repeatedly suffering with recurrent episodes of unhappiness or anxiety or any other neurotic problems then the outcome is less good. Instead of two out of five cases resolving within weeks only one out of five will get better. Such a finding is understandable if consideration is given to what is actually causing the problem or problems.

In the first instant (for new cases), it might be that an argument with a loved one over a lack of money or a dispute with an unruly teenager has led a distressed mother to become depressed and anxious. If the source of the problem is dealt with, or at least brought out into the open so that if can begin to be resolved, the symptoms experienced will usually go away.

However, if nothing is done to begin the process of resolution or nothing can be done to improve the situation then the sufferer will redevelop his or her symptoms again and again. And unless the source of the stress is dealt with, it is less and less likely that the unhappiness or anxiety will go away.

Looking again at figure 8, it is apparent that after about one year the number of patients getting better seems to have bottomed out. From that point, the outcomes are not clear. Some people will still get better, others will get worse and others still will remain at a constant state of unhappiness, or anxiety or neurosis.

Furthermore, if someone suffers a psychological insult then his or her ability to recover from the episode is also dependent upon other factors including the severity of the insult and the length of time the person has been subjected to the insult as well as the age at which the insult occurred.

The matter can be simplified by considering whether or not sufferers have what is often called 'the strength of character' to survive the index episode. Instead of strength of character, however, psychologists and psychiatrists would probably substitute the term *personality*.

Before looking at the outcome studies it is necessary to explore a little further the issue of insult mentioned above. Damaging or harmful episodes that may shape a person's character or personality can occur at anytime in life. The earlier the events occur the more likely there are to impact upon an individual's character.

Childhood abuse, particularly involving sexual activity, is an important factor in damaging the developing personality. The abuse may take many forms and have varying degrees of effect upon the life the victim may lead. But it is beyond doubt that rates of unhappiness, anxiety and other neurotic illnesses at least three or four times higher in sufferers of childhood abuse in women and at least double normal rates in men.

Previously, the issue of child abuse was one kept hidden in society, which probably allowed it to continue at shockingly high rates; some studies have recorded levels of up to 15% in girls and up to 10% in boys. However, in recent years the issue has received a much higher profile; health professionals are now given mandatory training about the matter and the general public have become aware of the issue through various campaigning organisations including ChildLine.[52]

With the key issues of personality or character and ideas of a predisposing vulnerability to the development of neurotic illness in mind, the outcomes of patients in the longer term will be considered. Much research has been done on the topic—especially with regard to depression—but there is no clear, straightforward general idea of how sufferers of neurotic illnesses fair in the long term. All that can be provided is a selection of the more important findings. These will illustrate how variable the future can be for such patients.

One longer-term study looking specifically at patients with depression, anxiety and the mixtures of the two conditions found that most sufferers over the years tend to move towards a state of more symptoms rather than less. That is those with anxiety symptoms alone moved to a mixed picture of anxiety and depression as did those with depression alone.

As has been discussed in Chapter One, symptoms from several different neurotic conditions tend to be present at the same time. For example, sufferers may have depressive symptoms along with anxiety symptoms, and patients with agoraphobia symptoms may have obsessional symptoms as well. In the context of the above study looking at long-term outcomes of anxiety and depression by themselves, this could be seen as rather short sighted. For as the patient's difficulties continue there is a tendency for them to develop more and more problems in a similar way to a snowball rolling down a hill getting bigger and bigger as it picks up more snow.[53]

That the tendency is for symptoms to increase in long-term sufferers of neurotic conditions helps both patient and doctor to appreciate one very important point: the longer the problem has been present the longer treatment—either psychological or pharmacological—will probably need to be given.

However, although most patients tend to develop more and more symptoms over time, there are probably fluctuations in the level of severity of these symptoms. One long-term study concluded that such sufferers of depression do indeed spend the majority of time at varying levels of misery. And researchers found that up to half of the patients were spending weeks at a time in mild states of unhappiness; of this group about a fifth were found to be suffering from a so-called subsyndromal illness, which essentially meant they were too well to warrant the label of 'disease'.[54]

The specific course that the illness will take is difficult to predict the first time that it occurs. Nevertheless, patients who have recovered completely having suffered from a period of depression or anxiety or any other type of neurotic illness are sort of primed psychologically to develop a recurrence of their symptoms if further distress comes along. Furthermore, people with more anxious or introverted characters or

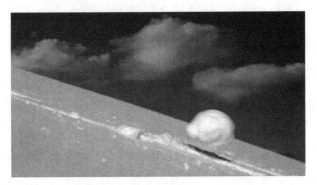

Figure 10. The Neurotic Snowball (Pimm 2013).

personalities are not only more susceptible initially to suffering from unhappiness, depression and other neurotic disorders, they are also prone to further breakdowns, which last longer and are more resistant to treatment or resolution.

A 46-year-old man became virtually housebound after the death of his long-term girlfriend. The couple had been together for more than 12 years when she developed breast cancer and died some 18 months after first complaining of pain. The loss of his partner was something felt very deeply but did not quite explain the complete psychological collapse seen in the patient. The situation became clearer when after several meetings the psychologist discovered that the patient's girlfriend had died on exactly the same date that his mother had passed away 20 years earlier with the same disease.

Another long-term outcome study reported that 85% of patients who recovered from an initial episode of major depression experienced a recurrence (see figure 11). And, in those who had remained free from any difficulties for at least five years after their first bout of unhappiness, nearly 60% had another episode of illness.

Bipolar Depression: Treatments and Outcomes

The concept of bipolar depression was introduced in Chapter 1. Essentially, it is depression occurring in someone who has a bipolar disorder but who has not yet had any episodes of mania or hypomania. Further, it might be that the episodes of mania or hypomania have been experienced by the patient but he or she simply did not come into contact with services at those times. This might have been because the person might have experienced the manic episodes as particularly enjoyable or exciting and, as such, not thought of them as being part of an illness or something out of the ordinary.

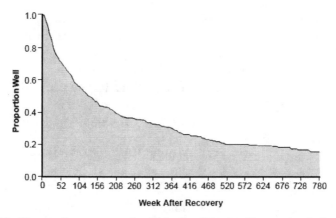

Figure 11. Time to Recurrence of an Episode of Further Depression in People Who Had Recovered from Their First Bout of Unhappiness (Mueller 1999).[55]

The importance of bipolar depression has only been recognised relatively recently, and it may account for as many as 10% of cases of people who were previously thought to simply have a straightforward depressive illness. This figure rises to 12.5% if episodes of hypomania or even subthreshold mania are counted as part of the mood disorder.

The importance of picking it up, or at least being aware of it, as early as possible relates to the need to alter treatment. Simply giving antidepressants is ineffective in such cases and may in fact make the situation worse. The recommended treatment is to combine the antidepressant with an antimanic agent (e.g., lithium, sodium valproate or an antipsychotic). Such treatment schedules require the supervision of a psychiatrist.

Conclusion

Health professionals, including hospital doctors and GPs, have long been criticised for their inability to spot, assess and treat depression as well as the other neurotic disorders. Their supposed inability to diagnose these common problems has led to the introduction of guidelines and protocols which have failed to produce the changes expected of them. The use of screening questionnaires has been criticised as unhelpful, and experts believe that they are unlikely to tackle the problems of how doctors deal with depression and the other neurotic conditions.

The whole process of trying to increase doctors ability to make sure that all sufferers are correctly identified has been seen as an unhelpful diversion from the more fundamental questions about the most efficient and effective way of organising and delivering care to such patients.

Up-to-date evidence points towards the use of a so-called chronic care model of management and treatment. Such a model would be multi-faceted and flexible so as to provide a level of support dependent upon the needs of the sufferer. This would necessitate particular close monitoring of the individual constantly over the whole course of the disease period. Treatments of any kind (psychological and pharmacological) could then be stepped up or stepped down depending upon need. Excessive or inappropriate treatments might thereby be avoided and the provision of the more intensive interventions would only be provided for those requiring them.

In an ideal world no one would become depressed or anxious! It is self evident that prevention is better than cure. The World Health Organisation (WHO) has produced much literature on evidence of the promotion of mental health and the prevention of illness. Recently under the mantra 'There is no health without mental health', the WHO has published a series of articles on the matter. It also gives a list of simple, effective interventions to show the value of such an approach. They include the following:

- Early childhood interventions (e.g., home visiting for pregnant women, pre-school psycho-social interventions, combined nutritional and psycho-social interventions in disadvantaged populations)
- Support to children (e.g., skills building programmes, child and youth development programmes)
- Socio-economic empowerment of women (e.g., improving access to education, microcredit schemes)
- Social support to old age populations (e.g., befriending initiatives, community and day centres for the aged)
- Programmes targeted at vulnerable groups, including minorities, indigenous people, migrants and people affected by conflicts and disasters (e.g., psycho-social interventions after disasters)
- Mental health promotion activities in schools (e.g., programmes supporting ecological changes in schools, child-friendly schools)
- Mental health interventions at work (e.g., stress prevention programmes)
- Housing policies (e.g., housing improvement)
- Violence prevention programmes (e.g., community policing initiatives)
- Community development programmes (e.g., 'Communities That Care' initiatives, integrated rural development)[56]

And Finally . . .

Neurosis and the other common mental disorders are ubiquitous. They come in different forms and combinations. They frequently resolve but often return. Sometimes they do not go away and grumble on and on.

Psychological and drug treatments often help but they are by no means a panacea.

To appreciate the situation fully, the problems must be seen in the context of the sufferer's past, present and future. Often they may simply represent an understandable, normal reaction and not an illness requiring medical or psychological interventions. And simple supportive networks— including both the traditional help of the extended family, the church and the local pub and the modern virtual interactions of social network and social media sites on the world wide web—are all that is required.

The internet has also impacted upon the way that patients find out about illnesses. They are no longer beholden to health professionals to provide them with details about diseases, diagnoses and drugs. Also, the web has enabled many patients with previously unrecognised conditions— particularly relevant in psychological and psychiatric disorders—to obtain specialist help.

Cheap, easily accessible air travel along with massive expansion of international trade has resulted in the need for health professionals from different countries and continents to communicate about shared care of patients. Further, such globalisation of illnesses has necessitated doctors dealing with patients from diverse backgrounds to be aware of important cultural differences. Such variations are seen not only in the manner patients present but also in the way that they may have been treated by the health professionals in other countries. These differences can be seen in both patients from developed and developing continents. For example, the

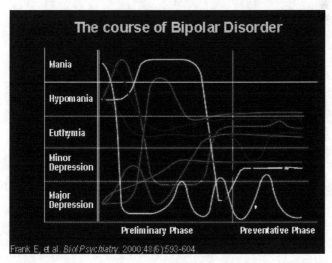

Figure 12. The Many and Varied Outcomes of Mood Disorders (Frank et al., 2000).[57]

city financier from New York may have been diagnosed with ADHD and depression by a doctor in the US who decided to use antidepressants and stimulant medication as the treatment. And from a developing country, patients suffering from a belief that they are possessed by evil spirits may in the UK be treated as a severe mental illness when in reality such ideas are culturally understandable.

Variations in professional practices are common in all specialities of medicine even within the UK itself. Differences are also seen between doctors operating and working in the private sector and their counterparts in the NHS. Alternative approaches to patients and treatments are particularly likely to occur in health professionals dealing with neurotic conditions.[58]

*   *   *

The last words in this journey through depression, anxiety and other neurotic conditions will be those of the Hungarian born medically trained psychoanalyst Michael Balint who explained:

> So the first principle should be: Never advise or reassure a patient before you have found out what the real problem is. More often than not, after the real problem has been brought to light, the patient will be able to solve it without the doctor's advice and reassurance.[59]

Stephen's Story: Part Seven

To end on a positive note would clearly have been ideal. And in Stephen's case the dramatic change that occurred following several months of him taking antidepressants and him attending regular sessions with the resident psychotherapist was a delight to behold.

The improvements were small to start with. On several occasions, Stephen was unsure whether he was actually feeling better. However, the words he used to describe his state were different, the colour returned to everything he said; black was no longer the predominant tinge.

And then one follow up appointment, about 3 months after his first assessment, he came into the room with a smile that made everything shine. He cracked a joke and explained that he was feeling a great deal better; he said he had feared he would never have experienced such positive emotions again when he was in the grips of his depression.

He remains well.

CHAPTER 4

Facts, Figures, Forms and Tables

The Professionals Involved

Counsellors — trained to administer counselling (see below).

Psychological wellbeing practitioners — a new type of counsellor specifically trained to deliver cognitive behavioural therapy to patients with common mental disorders in the primary care setting. They emerged from the 'Improving Access to Psychological Therapies' (IAPTs) service.

Psychologists — highly qualified therapists trained in psychology and then further educated to give a variety of different types of talking treatment to patients suffering from a wide range of mental disorders including depression, anxiety and other neurotic conditions and in some cases psychotic diseases as well. They are not medically qualified and are not licensed to prescribe drugs.

General Practitioners — medically qualified doctors who have specialised in medicine that is delivered in the primary care setting, i.e., in the community. They are experts at detecting disease and treating commonly occurring problems. They are often seen as the gatekeepers to services in the hospitals and in other secondary care settings.

Psychiatrists — medically qualified doctors who have specialised in psychological and psychiatric problems. They are often asked in what way they are different from psychologists. The answer is that psychiatrists are licensed to prescribe drugs and are skilled in differentiating psychologically generated physical problems from diseases which have an underlying pathology.

Psychotherapists — a generic term for anyone who is trained to deliver talking treatments to patients. They can be psychologists or doctors or both. Some doctors chose to extend their training in psychiatry by further developing skills to give psychological treatments to patients; they can be trained in any type of talking therapy including cognitive behavioural and psychodynamic (also known as psychoanalytic).

Community Psychiatric Nurses — nurses trained in looking after patients with psychiatric problems. They have usually spent time in psychiatric hospitals as part of the training but mainly operated in the community setting. They are usually attached to a community mental health team (see below).

The Psychiatric Services and Teams

Services are divided mainly between those at primary and secondary care level. Primary care means all those facilities available in the community, although this distinction has become rather blurred in recent years. It includes GPs and their surgeries and all those services they provide. Secondary care essentially means all services provided through hospitals and hospital outpatient departments.

Primary Care

At primary care level in the UK, expansion resulting from recent government policy has increased numbers of health care professionals involved in caring for patients with mental health difficulties. The so-called Improving Access to Psychological Therapies service (IAPTs) has led to a development of a new group of workers based in special community units and in GP surgeries.

Psychologists also work in General Practices at the primary care level. They may use a variety of different types of psychotherapy including CBT and psychoanalytical. They are more flexible in terms of the number of sessions they are able to offer and can when necessary see patients for several years.

Secondary Care

At secondary care level in the UK, help is provided by large multi-million pound NHS trusts. These are organisations that are essentially employed (or commissioned) by NHS budget holders to deliver care for patients with mental health difficulties. The Trust is composed of several different teams, which provide specific support and help aimed at meeting particular patients' needs.

The **Community Mental Health Team** (CMHT) will be staffed by individuals from several different disciplines including doctors, nurses and social workers. They may also have experts in helping patients find accommodation, work and sorting out problems with benefits. The CMHT is usually based in the community setting close to the general practitioner surgeries from where they receive most of their patients. The doctor (usually a consultant psychiatrist) heading the team will also be responsible for the care of patients when they are admitted to the local hospital. In some parts of the UK this model of service organisation has been scrapped in favour of an alternative arrangement; doctors are split in terms of those working in the community and those working in the hospital ward.

The **Assessment and Shared Care Team** (ASCT) is the name given to one of the teams operating in the community under an alternative method of service delivery. All patients are seen initially by the ASCT and from that point they may be directed to various other parts of the service depending upon their needs.

The **Rehabilitation and Recovery Team** (RRT) is another part of the alternative method of delivery of services. The RRT is responsible for the care of patients needing long term support and treatment.

The **Emergency Mental Health and Liaison Team**—all major hospitals will have a team of mental health professionals trained to provide care for patients attending Accident and Emergency units in general hospitals. They will assess patients needing psychiatric help. They may choose to refer the patients to another part of the service, discharge them home or admit them to the psychiatric ward.

Crisis Intervention Services provide interventions for patients in times of crises; they usually have a doctor attached to team but are mainly composed of psychologists, nurses and other experts trained in delivering talking treatments to patients in crises and in whom there has been detected a degree of risk in terms of suicide.

Psychological Therapies Services provide talking treatments for patients at secondary care level. The therapy is often long term and some cases may continue on for months or years. The department is staffed by both psychologists and psychiatrists skilled in talking treatments of several different types.

The **Assertive Outreach Team** is a team dedicated to the treatment of patients with long term difficulties usually schizophrenia. The service is available through referral from a psychiatrist at secondary care level and offers an enhanced package of help for patients who are often difficult to engage with and who carry an increased level of risk due to a criminal record or a history of violence.

The **Early Intervention and Early Detection Services** are provided for patients who are young (usually under 25 years) and who have recently been found to be suffering from schizophrenia. The Early Detection

Service aims to pick up people who either at high risk of developing the disease or who have shown early or prodromal symptoms.

Old Age Psychiatry—this service caters for patients over the age of 65 years who are suffering from mental illnesses; this includes individuals with dementias as well as more common psychiatric illnesses such as depression.

Other teams have been described by NHS organisations operating using alternative models. And the debate continues over which is the best and whether or not it should be uniformly adopted across the UK as a whole.

The Psychiatric Assessment

Psychiatrists and other mental health professionals will usually undertake an assessment of the sufferer. Patients are commonly surprised (pleasantly in most cases) at just how long the initial meeting is; in psychiatric outpatients the first assessment is usually about an hour. They are used to only having a few minutes to see their GPs. They sometimes fear they will not know what to say for the whole session and it is then up to the doctor or other health professional to reassure them that he or she will direct the proceedings to a certain extent. In some circumstances sufferers are so desperate to tell their story that the doctor may have to interrupt and direct them to specific areas so that he or she may obtain a fuller, broad brush picture of the problem rather than focussing on one particular aspect.

Often during the assessment process, patients will ask why a particular question is relevant to their problem. Therefore, in an attempt to enlighten the enquiring sufferer, all the sections of the formulaic psychiatric interview will be discussed and their relevance particularly to depression, anxiety and the other neurotic conditions explained. The sections of the interview are as follows:

1. The **presenting complaint** — here the interviewer will record usually verbatim exactly what the patient has come to see the doctor about. It is best to use the sufferer's own words so that any professional reading through the notes in the future will be able to gain a clearer picture of how the patient expressed himself or herself. For example, a doctor might record the problems as: 'I am having dark thoughts' or 'I get these pains in my fingers' or 'I feel depressed' and so on.
2. The **history of the presenting complaint** will record details about the presenting complaints including when the problems started, how often they occur, and whether or not they have been getting worse, or staying the same or even getting better. It is particularly difficult to get a clear

history of a patient's level of happiness or unhappiness—a task made harder when the matter has been troublesome for many years. Often in such situations it is simply best to record the patient's story and wait to see how things develop over the forthcoming days, weeks or months, and then try to put what was said at the initial interview in context of what has emerged.

The additional aim of the history of the presenting complaint section is to confirm or dismiss the presence or absence of additional symptoms in an effort to develop a working diagnosis. For example, if the patient states he or she is depressed, then the doctor is duty bound to ask about other symptoms of depression, i.e., energy levels, mood levels, suicidal thoughts, appetite, sleep problems and so on. Or if the patient has recurrent nightmares or flashbacks about an upsetting situation, the doctor should ask further questions about avoidance of certain places and thoughts and other symptoms of post traumatic stress disorder.

3. The **past psychiatric history** — previous contacts with psychiatric or psychological services will also be questioned. The doctor will ask whether the patient has been admitted to hospital before with psychiatric problems in an attempt to gauge the severity of the patient's past difficulties. Further, if the patient has been seen by a psychologist and received previous talking therapy treatment it might have a bearing upon which level of treatment might be appropriate for the current problem; the same goes for past drugs used.

4. The **past medical history** may be very relevant in terms of why he or she has developed a psychiatric problem. Various medical conditions can lead to mental health difficulties.

5. The **family history** may be important in terms of searching for elements of psychiatric illnesses that can be inherited. Also, it might be relevant since a patient may have experienced a particularly disturbing upbringing because of a parent was suffering from a mental illness.

6. The **personal history** — the record of the patient's past, beginning from birth to the present day, will also be important as it might give clues to the reason why such a problem has developed. The personal history also gives indications of the patient's personality or character which is helpful to the assessor; often the patient's character will determine which type of neurotic condition or conditions will develop later in life.

7. The **social history** — this will include a record of the patient's current housing situation, their job, their relationships (including sexual ones) and their financial situation.

8. **Drug history** — the patient's use of drugs and alcohol will be recorded

9. **Forensic history** — the patient's previous experiences with the criminal justice system will be recorded.
10. **Medication history** — a record of all medications prescribed (and not prescribed) is made.
11. **Personality, hobbies and religion** — enquiring about the patient's thoughts as to their own character or what their friends might think is their character can be helpful. Also, a record of hobbies and other activities may indicate the type of life the patient lives. Religion and religious beliefs may be important.
12. The **mental state examination** — this is really a checklist for the assessing doctor to make sure particularly important facts have been formally recorded.
    (a) Appearance and behaviour
    (b) Speech
    (c) Mood including affect
    (d) Thought — form and content
    (e) Perceptions
    (f) Insight — expressed wishes, expectations
13. **Risk** — here a formal risk assessment is recorded.
14. **Formulation** — here a summary of the case is given with a more analytical look at how the individual's difficulties have arisen.
15. **Outcome** — the planned outcome of the assessment is recorded.

Manuals, Questionnaires and Scales

ICD 10 and DSM IV

The International Classification of Diseases (ICD) 10 is the diagnostic manual mainly used by psychiatrists in the UK and is published by the World Health Organisation; the ICD-11 is due to be published in the near future. The Americans use the Diagnostic and Statistical Manual of Mental Disorders (DSM) IV to classify psychiatric disorders. DSM 5 [*sic*] has recently been published. DSM IV and DSM 5 differ from the ICD-10 because they allow diagnoses along several different axes. Clinical disorders are placed on Axis I and other disorders including personality disorders and mental retardation are placed on Axis II. Axis III describes physical illness contributing to the emotional problems, Axis IV refers to the level of social functioning at a designated point (e.g., at admission or discharge) and Axis V refers to stressors in the previous six months. The DSM justifies axes because 'placing [a disorder] on a separate axis ensures that consideration will be given to the possible presence of problems that might otherwise be overlooked when attention is directed to the usually more florid Axis I disorders'.

The criteria for depression of the DSM IV will be given below for comparison with the ICD 10 and because they were used in the construction of the PHQ-9.

ICD-10 Diagnostic Criteria for Depression: Mild, Moderate, Severe

The ICD-10 criteria share some of the symptoms in the PHQ-9 but they allow the physician to categorise the patient more specifically. The initial classification in the F32 section of the manual describes three varieties - namely mild (F32.0), moderate (F32.1) and severe (F32.2 and F32.3).

The three *core* symptoms (below) are listed as the core problems of the disorder:

1. Depressed mood
2. Loss of interest and enjoyment (also known as anhedonia).
3. Reduced energy leading to increased fatiguability and diminished activity

Other common symptoms are:

1. Reduced concentration and attention
2. Reduced self-esteem and self-confidence
3. Ideas of guilt and unworthiness (even in a mild type of episode)
4. Bleak and pessimistic views of the future
5. Ideas or acts of self-harm or suicide
6. Diminished sleep
7. Diminished appetite

For the three grades of severity (mild, moderate and severe), a duration of at least **two weeks** is usually required for diagnosis.

The manual further explains that some of the above symptoms may be marked and develop characteristic features widely regarded as having special clinical significance. It goes on to explain that the most common of these so-called somatic symptoms are:

1. Loss of interest or pleasure in activities that are normally enjoyable
2. Lack of emotional reactivity to normally pleasurable surroundings and events

3. Waking in the morning 2 hours or more before the usual time
4. Depression worse in the morning
5. Objective evidence of definite psychomotor retardation or agitation (remarked on or reported by other people
6. Marked loss of appetite
7. Weight loss (often defined as 5% or more of body weight in the past month)
8. Marked loss of libido

The somatic **syndrome** is defined as being present only when about **four** of the above symptoms are definitely present.

Mild Depression

This is defined by the presence of at least **two** of the **core** symptoms (listed above) being present with at least **two** of the **other** (listed above) for at least two weeks. An individual with a mild depressive episode is usually distressed by the symptoms and has some difficulty in continuing with ordinary work and social activities, but will probably not cease to function completely. Mild depression is classified further with regard to the presence or absence of the somatic syndrome (note again, for this to be present, four of the somatic symptoms need to be seen).

Moderate Depression

This is defined by the presence of at least **two** of the **core** symptoms being present with at least **three (preferably four)** of the **other** symptoms for at least two weeks. Moderate depression is classified further with regard to the presence or absence of the somatic syndrome.

Severe Depression

This is defined by the presence of all **three** of the **core** symptoms with at least **four** of the **other** symptoms, some of which should be of severe intensity. In a severe depressive episode the sufferers usually show considerable distress or agitation, unless retardation is a marked feature. Loss of self-esteem or feelings of uselessness or guilt are likely to be prominent and suicide is a distinct danger. It is presumed that somatic syndrome is almost always present in a severe depressive episode.

Severe depression is classified further with regard to the presence or absence of **psychotic** symptoms. If delusions, hallucinations or a depressive stupor are present then the patient should be thought of as psychotic. The delusions usually involve ideas of sin, poverty or imminent disasters. Auditory hallucinations or olfactory hallucinations are usually defamatory or accusatory voices or of rotting filth or decomposing flesh.

Core symptoms	Other symptoms	Somatic symptoms*
Depressed mood	Reduced concentration and attention	Loss of interest or pleasure in activities that are normally enjoyable
Loss of interest and enjoyment (also known as anhedonia)	Reduced self-esteem and self-confidence	Lack of emotional reactivity to normally pleasurable surroundings and events
Reduced energy leading to increased fatigability and diminished activity	Ideas of guilt and unworthiness (even in a mild type of episode)	Waking in the morning 2 hours or more before the usual time
	Bleak and pessimistic views of the future	Depression worse in the morning
	Ideas or acts of self-harm or suicide	Objective evidence of definite psychomotor retardation or agitation (remarked on or reported by other people)
	Diminished sleep	Marked loss of appetite
	Diminished appetite	Weight loss (often defined as 5% or more of body weight in the past month) Marked loss of libido

Figure 13. Symptoms Present in Depression.
* The somatic syndrome is defined as being present only when at least four of the above somatic symptoms are definitely present.

DSM-IV Diagnostic Criteria for Depression

The DSM-IV criteria for depression are included because they are similar to those of the PHQ-9. The diagnosis of major depressive episode is used if the patient has:

Five (or more) of the following symptoms have been present during the same **2-week** period and represent a change from previous functioning. **At least one** of the symptoms is either:

1. Depressed mood or
2. Loss of interest or pleasure

Note: Do not include symptoms that are clearly due to a general medical condition, or mood-incongruent delusions or hallucinations. The first two are an expansion of the two listed above and as stated before, one of these has to be included in the five or more.

1. Depressed mood most of the day, nearly every day, as indicated by either subjective report (e.g., feels sad or empty) or observation made by

others (e.g., appears tearful). Note: In children and adolescents, there can be irritable mood

2. Markedly diminished interest or pleasure in all, or almost all, activities most of the day, nearly every day (as indicated by either subjective account or observation made by others)
3. Significant weight loss when not dieting or weight gain (e.g., a change of more than 5% of body weight in a month), or decrease or increase in appetite nearly every day. Note: In children, consider failure to make expected weight gain.
4. Insomnia or hypersomnia nearly every day
5. Psychomotor agitation or retardation nearly every day (observable by others, not merely subjective feelings of restlessness or being slowed down)
6. Fatigue or loss of energy nearly every day
7. Feelings of worthlessness or excessive or inappropriate guilt (which may be delusional) nearly every day (not merely self-reproach or guilt about being sick)
8. Diminished ability to think or concentrate, or indecisiveness, nearly every day (either by subjective account or as observed by others)
9. Recurrent thoughts of death (not just fear of dying), recurrent suicidal ideation without a specific plan, or a suicide attempt or specific plan for committing suicide

The DSM-IV goes further to classify the major depressive episode as being *melancholic* or *non-melancholic*. The diagnosis of melancholic depends upon the presence of important additional symptoms including complete loss of pleasure in virtually all activities, lack of reactivity, a distinct almost painful quality to the depressed mood, motor slowing, agitation, marked disturbance of sleep and appetite and diurnal variation of symptoms. Guilt may be excessive or even psychotic.

NICE Guidelines

Guidelines on how to treat depression and anxiety have also been produced by NICE.

The treatment recommendations for depression are based upon clinical ICD-10 diagnoses and adopt a so-called 'stepped care' approach (see figure 14). The treatments for depression fall into four main categories:

1. Watchful waiting — essentially observation
2. Self-help treatments — which can either be done by the patient alone or guided by a primary care mental health worker
3. Psychological treatments — these are in two main categories; in essence short or long term
4. Medication

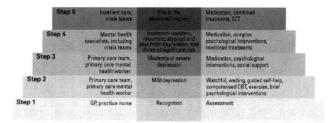

Figure 14. The Stepped-Care Model.

The basis of treatment protocols requires an accurate diagnosis. Once the problem is clear then the appropriate treatment can be prescribed. This can be simply summarised as:

Mild depression — watchfully wait and/or self-help and/or computerised psychological therapy and/or brief psychological interventions
Moderate depression — antidepressant and/or psychological (talking) therapy
Severe depression — complex psychological interventions and/or antidepressant or other medications and/or ECT.

The treatment options for anxiety (including generalised anxiety disorder and panic disorder with or without agoraphobia) as outlined in the NICE guidelines are essentially, antidepressants and/or self-help and/or guided self-help and/or psychological treatments. The only other major point to note in the NICE guidelines for anxiety disorders is that drugs like benzodiazepines and other anxiolytics are not recommended.

Questionnaires

PHQ-2

The screening questions of the Patient Health Questionnaire—2 (PHQ-2) have been shown to be both sensitive and specific. They are:

1. Over the last two weeks, how often have you been bothered by little interest or pleasure in doing things?

and

2. Over the last two weeks, how often have you been feeling down depressed or hopeless?

A 'yes' to either of the questions can be considered a positive test result and should prompt further examination.

PHQ-2

Over the past two weeks, how often have you been bothered by any of the
following problems?
    Little interest or pleasure in doing things.
    0 = Not at all
    1 = Several days
    2 = More than half the days
    3 = Nearly every day
    Feeling down, depressed, or hopeless.
    0 = Not at all
    1 = Several days
    2 = More than half the days
    3 = Nearly every day

    Total point score: _____

Figure 15. Example of PHQ-2 Question.

PHQ-9

The Patient Health Questionnaire—9 (PHQ-9) has become the instrument
of choice in recent years for GPs once they suspect a depressive disorder.
This is an easy to use questionnaire, which the patient fills in. It scores
each of the nine criteria for depression found in the DSM-IV as '0' (not at
all), '1' (on several days), '2' (more than half the days), '3' (nearly every
day) depending on whether the patient has been 'bothered' by a list of nine
problems over the previous two weeks.

The questionnaire's validity has been assessed against an independent
structured mental health professional interview. A PHQ-9 score of greater
than or equal to 10 had a sensitivity of 88% and a specificity of 88% for
major depression.

A score on the PHQ-9 of 0-4 represents no disease, 10-14 moderate
depression, 15-19 moderately severe depression and 20-27 severe
disease.

The Hospital Anxiety and Depression Scale (HADS)

The HADS is a commonly used scale to assess patients' anxiety and
depression.[60] It is a self-report questionnaire which is well recognised as
being reliable and valid in the diagnosis of both anxiety and depression. In
practice it would be used in the assessment of patients by more specialised
practitioners, e.g., psychiatrists and psychologists. It is used both before
and after therapy or treatment in an effort to establish whether the patient
has improved or not.

PATIENT HEALTH QUESTIONNAIRE-9 (PHQ-9)

Over the last 2 weeks, how often have you been bothered by any of the following problems? (Use "✔" to indicate your answer)	Not at all	Several days	More than half the days	Nearly every day
1. Little interest or pleasure in doing things	0	1	2	3
2. Feeling down, depressed, or hopeless	0	1	2	3
3. Trouble falling or staying asleep, or sleeping too much	0	1	2	3
4. Feeling tired or having little energy	0	1	2	3
5. Poor appetite or overeating	0	1	2	3
6. Feeling bad about yourself — or that you are a failure or have let yourself or your family down	0	1	2	3
7. Trouble concentrating on things, such as reading the newspaper or watching television	0	1	2	3
8. Moving or speaking so slowly that other people could have noticed? Or the opposite — being so fidgety or restless that you have been moving around a lot more than usual	0	1	2	3
9. Thoughts that you would be better off dead or of hurting yourself in some way	0	1	2	3

FOR OFFICE CODING ___0___ + _____ + _____ + _____

=Total Score: _____

If you checked off any problems, how difficult have these problems made it for you to do your work, take care of things at home, or get along with other people?

Not difficult at all	Somewhat difficult	Very difficult	Extremely difficult
☐	☐	☐	☐

Figure 16. PHQ-9 Questionnaire.

Generalised Anxiety Disorder (GAD)

A self-report questionnaire used in the diagnosis and assessment of generalised anxiety disorder.[61] It is commonly used by specialists involved in treatment of anxiety and may be employed to assess patients before and after care.

Adult ADHD

The diagnostic interview for ADHD in adults (DIVA) is a questionnaire filled in by the health care professional involved in the care of patients with or with suspected adult ADHD.[62] It has two main sections, the first looking

Hospital Anxiety and Depression Scale (HADS)

Patients are asked to choose one response from the four given for each interview. They should give an immediate response and be dissuaded from thinking too long about their answers. The questions relating to anxiety are marked "A", and to depression "D". The score for each answer is given in the right column. Instruct the patient to answer how it currently describes their feelings.

A	I feel tense or 'wound up':	
	Most of the time	3
	A lot of the time	2
	From time to time, occasionally	1
	Not at all	0

D	I still enjoy the things I used to enjoy:	
	Definitely as much	0
	Not quite so much	1
	Only a little	2
	Hardly at all	3

A	I get a sort of frightened feeling as if something awful is about to happen:	
	Very definitely and quite badly	3
	Yes, but not too badly	2
	A little, but it doesn't worry me	1
	Not at all	0

D	I can laugh and see the funny side of things:	
	As much as I always could	0
	Not quite so much now	1
	Definitely not so much now	2
	Not at all	3

Figure 17. HADS Anxiety and Depression Scale Questionnaire. (Continued)

A	Worrying thoughts go through my mind:	
	A great deal of the time	3
	A lot of the time	2
	From time to time, but not too often	1
	Only occasionally	0

D	I feel cheerful:	
	Not at all	3
	Not often	2
	Sometimes	1
	Most of the time	0

A	I can sit at ease and feel relaxed:	
	Definitely	0
	Usually	1
	Not Often	2
	Not at all	3

D	I feel as if I am slowed down:	
	Nearly all the time	3
	Very often	2
	Sometimes	1
	Not at all	0

A	I get a sort of frightened feeling like 'butterflies' in the stomach:	
	Not at all	0
	Occasionally	1
	Quite Often	2
	Very Often	3

Figure 17. HADS Anxiety and Depression Scale Questionnaire.   (Continued)

D	I have lost interest in my appearance:	
	Definitely	3
	I don't take as much care as I should	2
	I may not take quite as much care	1
	I take just as much care as ever	0

A	I feel restless as I have to be on the move:	
	Very much indeed	3
	Quite a lot	2
	Not very much	1
	Not at all	0

D	I look forward with enjoyment to things:	
	As much as I ever did	0
	Rather less than I used to	1
	Definitely less than I used to	2
	Hardly at all	3

A	I get sudden feelings of panic:	
	Very often indeed	3
	Quite often	2
	Not very often	1
	Not at all	0

D	I can enjoy a good book or radio or TV program:	
	Often	0
	Sometimes	1
	Not often	2
	Very seldom	3

Figure 17. HADS Anxiety and Depression Scale Questionnaire. (Continued)

Scoring (add the As = Anxiety. Add the Ds = Depression). The norms below will give you an idea of the level of Anxiety and Depression.	
0-7 = Normal	
8-10 = Borderline abnormal	
11-21 = Abnormal	

Figure 17. HADS Anxiety and Depression Scale Questionnaire.

for symptoms relating to an inability to concentrate and the second looking mainly for problems of over activity.

Each question seeks to find out whether the symptoms commonly found in ADHD are present at the time of the assessment and also if the person suffered from the same difficulties in childhood.

Conclusion

Health care services set up for the assessment, treatment and management of patients with mental and psychological difficulties are numerous and varied. They include psychiatric wards, outpatient departments and specialist multi-disciplinary teams. Most professionals will assess patients using structured, formal interviews. They may also use recognised scientifically tested questionnaires to undertake further investigation of the patient. Caution needs to be exercised in the use of such questionnaires since they may produce misleading results. They might conclude that someone has a particular disorder incorrectly or they might indeed miss the illness completely. Ideally, they should be seen only as an adjunct to the thorough assessment, confirming the presence or absence of a suspected problem.

In some cases the questionnaires are used as a screening tool where they are given indiscriminately to anyone presenting to a doctor or health care professional in the hope that any illness like depression or anxiety may be picked up and treated. The use of questionnaires in screening is fraught with difficulties particularly that of over diagnosis.

Endnotes

1. Prochaska, JO, Norcross, JC; DiClemente, CC. *Changing for Good: The Revolutionary Program That Explains the Six Stages of Change and Teaches You How to Free Yourself from Bad Habits.* New York: W. Morrow. 1994.
2. Stigma is the reaction of society to a particular situation. The reaction can be felt by the individual or can be expressed by members of the society to the person with the stigmatizing problem.
3. Even though the situation has arisen at the same time as the woman's period, it is not possible to say that it is the hormones that have caused the mental health difficulty. There is likely to be some other step or pathway involved in the production of the depressive symptoms, i.e., an intermediate hormone as yet unidentified.
4. In the context of the current understanding of how mental illness develops, such a statement is incorrect. Everything must ultimately come from within before it can be experienced; the external environment is perceived by the sensory organs, which then impacts upon the biology of the sufferer to produce the biological state that is described or felt as unhappiness or any other emotional state.
5. This allows compulsory admission into a psychiatric unit for assessment and treatment of a psychiatric disorder if a person is thought to be at serious risk of harm to self or others due to mental illness.
6. The ideas about personality and its traits were first described in psychology by Hans Eysenck. His wife Sybil was very much involved with the concepts and is credited jointly with her husband for devising the Personality Questionnaire.
7. Melfi C.A, Croghan T.W, Hanna M.P,. Robinson R.L. Racial variation in antidepressant treatment in a Medicaid population. Journal of Clinical Psychiatry. 2000 Jan; 61(1):16-21
8. Delusions are defined as fixed, false beliefs that are unshakably held by the sufferer or sufferers that are out of keeping with the individual's social and cultural background.
9. Hallucinations are defined as perceptions without objects.
10. Disordered thoughts are those that have not coherence or logical structure to them.
11. Insight is usually gauged simply on the individual's ability to accept they are ill.
12. Precontemplative is a term coined by Prochaska and DiClemente in their landmark text *The Transtheoretical Approach: Crossing the traditional boundaries of therapy.* (1985).

13. Also known as the Emergency Room.
14. The term clinically depressed implies that the condition has reached the level whereby a doctor would classify the patient as ill.
15. The story goes that if someone talks about suicidal ideas initially then that is not too worrying; the fear is that when they stop talking about them it indicates that they have either got better or they have had a vague idea that has crystallised into a clear plan of how they might take their own life but do not want to tell anyone for fear that they might be stopped or detained in a mental institution.
16. Anxiety is given the more wordy, if not worthy, title of Generalised Anxiety Disorder (GAD) by clinicians.
17. Animals that chew the cud are vegetarians who have to regurgitate plant foodstuffs to give them a second grinding in the mouth.
18. Freud used the term *hysteria* to refer to situations when patients suffered physical problems that had no underlying pathology. He expanded the idea by stating that such patients had gained in some way from their problems; primary gain was the benefit the patient had by not having to suffer his or her psychiatric difficulties like depression or anxiety, and secondary gain referred to the benefit the patient had by not having to perform a particularly activity in his or her daily life.
19. 'Psychologically unexplained symptoms' (PUSs) is a phrase constructed by this author.
20. Launer, John, Medically Unexplored Stories, Postgraduate Medical Journal 2009; 85:503-504.
21. The *unconscious mind* is another term attributed to Freud; essentially it refers to those memories that are inaccessible unless specific techniques are adopted. The use of dream interpretation, hypnosis and 'free association' in therapy are some of the methods Freud advocated using to access the unconscious.
22. The International Classification of Diseases version 10 is a manual produced by the World Health Organisation to classify and aid in the diagnosis of diseases.
23. Parkes, C.M., & Weiss, R. (1983). *Recovery from Bereavement*. New York: Basic Books.
24. After Heyman I, Mataix-Cols D, Fineberg NA. Obsessive-compulsive disorder. BMJ 2006; 333:424-429.
25. The so called common mental disorders (CMDs) are depression alone, anxiety (generalised anxiety disorder) alone and mixed anxiety and depressive disorder (MADD).
26. Although an elevated mood is the more classic or typical finding in the manic or hypomanic patient, it may be that this euphoria is either replaced by or accompanied by a degree of irritability or 'touchiness'.
27. A review by Sophia Frangou gives an excellent outline of the current understanding on the subject of bipolar depression (Advances in Psychiatric Treatment (2005), vol. 11, 28-37).
28. Sigmund Freud described various levels of awareness of memories for past

events. Those easily accessed were stored in the conscious mind, those need-ing a trigger of some sort were in the pre-conscious and those requiring special techniques to either get at them or give indications of them were hid-den in the unconscious. The various techniques required involved analysis of dreams or slips or the tongue or so-called free association while lying on the couch.

29. Compliance refers to whether the patient chooses to do what the doctor has recommended. It is well recognized that up to 40% of patients never take pre-scribed medications correctly either at the correct dose or for the right length of time.

30. *Illness behavior* is a term first coined and investigated by David Mechanic who identified 10 variables that influence patients' actions when they become sick. These include whether or not the disease is visible, the perceived serious-ness of the symptoms, the amount of disruption the symptoms cause and the tolerance threshold of the person.

31. Talcott Parsons described the concept of the 'sick role' in 1951 which gives people who are ill certain rights and responsibilities.

32. Balint, Michael. (1964). *The Doctor, His Patient and the Illness* (2nd ed.). London: Pitman Medical Publishing.

33. The term *secondary care* refers to any part of the health service that is not primary care; this may be a hospital, an outpatient clinic or a specialist unit.

34. Unhappiness specifically brought about in the winter months when there is a lack of natural daylight has been called seasonal affective disorder (SAD). The syndrome has provoked much debate among sufferers and health profes-sionals alike.

35. Veale, *Advances in Psychiatric Treatment* (2008) 14: 29-36

36. Medications are classified by their mechanism of action. They are named according to their chemical composition. But they are also given a trade name or brand name under which they are marketed by the manufacturer.

37. Buproprion is classified as both an antidepressant and adjunct treatment to help people quit smoking.

38. Lithium carbonate is a naturally occurring salt that is commonly used to treat bipolar disorder.

39. Tryptophan is an essential amino acid.

40. Williams, C. J. (2001a) *Overcoming Depression: A Five Areas Approach*. London: Arnold.

41. The quotation marks serve to illustrate language commonly used by doctors. They do not represent this doctor's recommendation.

42. Cyclothymia describes a condition that resembles bipolar disorder, with the alternation of (hypo) manic phases and depressive periods, but to a lesser extent than bipolar disorder. The highs and lows are not extreme enough to fit the diagnostic criteria for bipolar disorder. It is an exaggerated form of the normal variations in mood of an individual.

43. Dysthymia refers to a state of chronic low mood, which does not fit the criteria for a major depressive disorder. Individuals with dysthymia can suffer consid-

erably despite the apparent lack of significance implicit in the diagnostic label.

44. Many chemicals exist in two different forms called isomers. These forms are labelled left and right; they are mirror images of one another. They are the same chemical formulae but different structurally.

45. A formulation of the issue aims to link the patient's previous experiences and difficulties to the current problem.

46. Layard, R. (2006) The case for psychological treatment centres. *British Medical Journal,* 332, 1030–2

47. Attachment theory relates to the ties between a child and its mother.

48. Kirsch, I., Deacon, B. J., Huedo-Medina, T. B., Scoboria, A., Moore, T. J., & Johnson, B. T. (2008). Initial severity and antidepressant benefits: a meta-analysis of data submitted to the food and drug administration, PLoS Medicine, 5(2), e45 EP

49. 'Cognitive behavioural therapy for major psychiatric disorder: does it really work? A meta-analytical review of well-controlled trials' by Lynch *et al.* (2009)

50. Reducing dependency, increasing opportunity: options for the future of welfare to work. An independent report to the Department for Work and Pensions was written by David Freud (2007). He is the great grandson of Sigmund Freud.

51. Markov models were used by Professor Scott B. Patten to demonstrate outcomes of incident cases.

52. http://www.childline.org.uk/Pages/Home.aspx. This is an organisation originally set up by British TV celebrity Esther Rantzen in 1986.

53. The concept of the neurotic snowball was first described by the author in 2011 during a lecture series delivered to GPs.

54. Judd LL, Akiskal HS, Maser JD, Zeller PJ, Endicott J, Coryell W, Paulus MP, Kunovac JL, Leon AC, Mueller TI, Rice JA, Keller MB. Major depressive disorder: a prospective study of residual subthreshold depressive symptoms as predictor of rapid relapse. J Affect Disord. 1998 Sep;50(2-3):97-108.

55. Timothy I. Mueller, M.D.; Andrew C. Leon, Ph.D.; Martin B. Keller, M.D.; David A. Solomon, M.D.; Jean Endicott, Ph.D.; William Coryell, M.D.; Meredith Warshaw, M.S.S., M.A.; Jack D. Maser, Ph.D. Recurrence After Recovery From Major Depressive Disorder During 15 Years of Observational Follow-Up. Am J Psychiatry 1999;156:1000-1006

56. The interested reader is advised to follow the link below to the WHO website: http://www.who.int/topics/mental_health/en/

57. Frank E, Swartz HA, Kupfer DJ. Interpersonal and social rhythm therapy: Managing the chaos of bipolar disorder. Biol Psychiatry. 2000 Sep 15;48(6):593-604.

58. The reasons involve the poorly defined nature of the conditions and the difficulty in separating them from normal experience as well as the limited efficacy of the treatments.

59. Michael Balint's famous book *The Doctor, His Patient and the Illness* was published first in 1957 and updated in 1964 emphasised the importance of the relationship between physicians and their patients.

60. Zigmond, A. S. & Snaith, R. P. (1983) The Hospital Anxiety and Depression Scale. Acta Psychiatrica Scandinavica, 67, 361-370.
61. Spitzer RL, Kroenke K, Williams JB, et al A brief measure for assessing generalized anxiety disorder: the GAD-7. Arch Intern Med. 2006 May 22;166(10):1092-7.
62. Kooij JJS, Francken MH. DIVA 2.0. Diagnostic Interview Voor ADHD in Adults bij volwassenen. DIVA 2.0. Diagnostic Interview ADHD in Adults. DIVA Foundation, 2010.

Index

A
adjustment disorder, 27, 45ff, 51
adult ADHD, 64, 119ff
alcohol misuse, 21ff, 67ff, 71, 78, 94
antidepressants, 15, 18, 71ff, 75ff, 83, 84, 87, 94

B
binge / binge drinking, 15, 24, 67
bipolar disorder, 21, 52ff, 64, 82, 93, 94, 102, 103

C
childhood abuse, 44, 45, 100
community psychiatric nurse / CPN, 62, 108
consultation, 18, 21, 23, 25, 56, 59ff, 65
counsellor / counselling, 19, 25, 33, 62, 80, 86ff, 95, 107
cyberchondriasis, 64
cyclothymia, 82, 127

D
delusions, 20, 29, 85, 114, 115, 125
dementia, 43, 110
DIVA, 55, 119
dysthymia, 32, 56, 82

E
EEG, 44
endogenous, 7ff, 72
extrovert, 14, 22
Eysenck, Hans, 15, 16, 112, 125

F
flashbacks, 40, 48, 111
Freud, Sigmund, 20, 43, 57, 92, 126, 128

G
goodness of fit, 14

H
hallucinations, 20, 43ff, 79, 85, 114, 115, 125

I
ICD, 46, 112, 113, 116
internet, 56, 64, 66, 69, 105
introvert, 14, 17, 22, 101

L
lithium, 76, 83, 103, 127

M
mania / manic, 21, 27, 40, 52, 53, 65, 83, 102, 103, 126

medically unexplained symptoms / MUS, 42, 45, 62
methylphenidate, 85
MIND, 87
MRI scan, 10, 42, 44

N
neurotic / neuroticism, 14ff, 20ff, 27, 32, 36, 40, 48ff, 58, 62, 64, 66ff, 70ff, 82, 85ff, 94, 97ff

O
obsessive compulsive disorder / OCD, 27, 40, 52
outcome, 3, 4, 7, 49, 83, 93, 97ff, 112
over valued ideas, 29, 36, 51

P
pain, 24, 34, 40ff, 69, 82, 102, 110
panic attacks / disorder, 4, 14, 27, 37ff, 76, 79, 117
perpetuating factor, 17
personality, 13ff, 21, 32, 47, 54, 61, 64, 91ff, 100, 101, 111, 112, 125
phobia / phobic, 20, 21, 27, 36ff, 50, 52, 78, 88, 95, 101, 117
pilates, 71
placebo, 86, 94, 95
precipitating factor, 17
pre contemplative, 24, 125
predisposing factor, 17, 101
pregabalin, 82

prognosis (see also outcomes), 36, 98
psychoanalysis / psychoanalyst, 43, 68, 91, 92, 106, 108
psychoticism, 16

R
risk, 11, 30, 31, 53, 69, 74, 92, 95, 96, 109
ruminations, 50, 78, 99

S
schizophrenia, 21, 27, 43, 94, 109
self harm, 14, 28, 30, 92, 113
snowball, 71, 101, 102
stepped care, 116, 117
stigma, 3, 25, 60, 97, 125
stress, 9, 40, 46, 48, 56, 61, 66, 67, 71, 78, 100, 104, 113
subsyndromal, 7, 52, 53, 101

T
tai chi, 71
timeline, 65
tsunami, 48

U
unconscious, 45, 57, 92, 126, 127

W
World Health Organisation / WHO, 27, 104, 112, 126

Y
yoga, 71